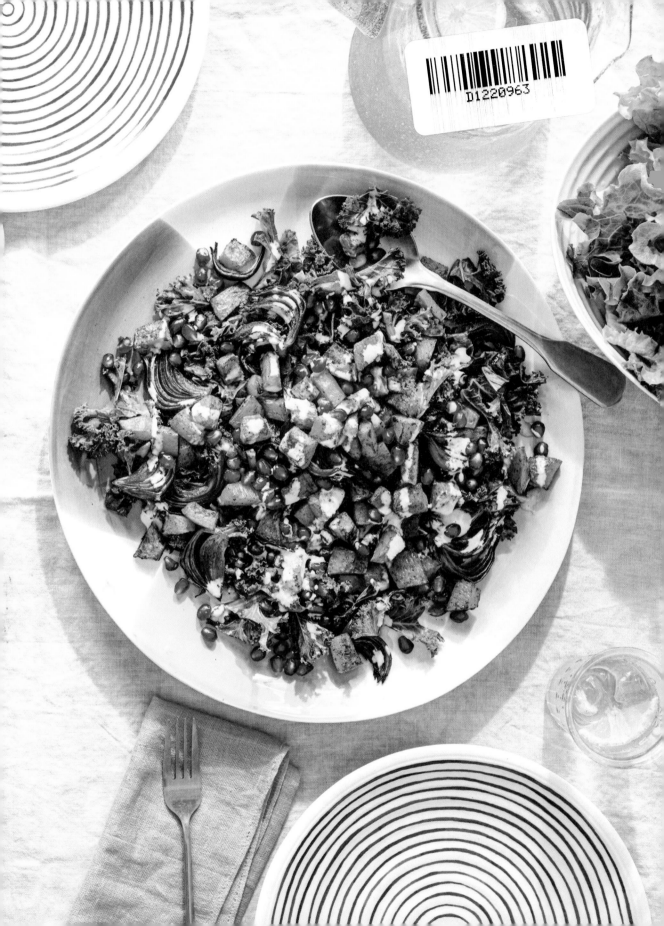

Slimming
EATS

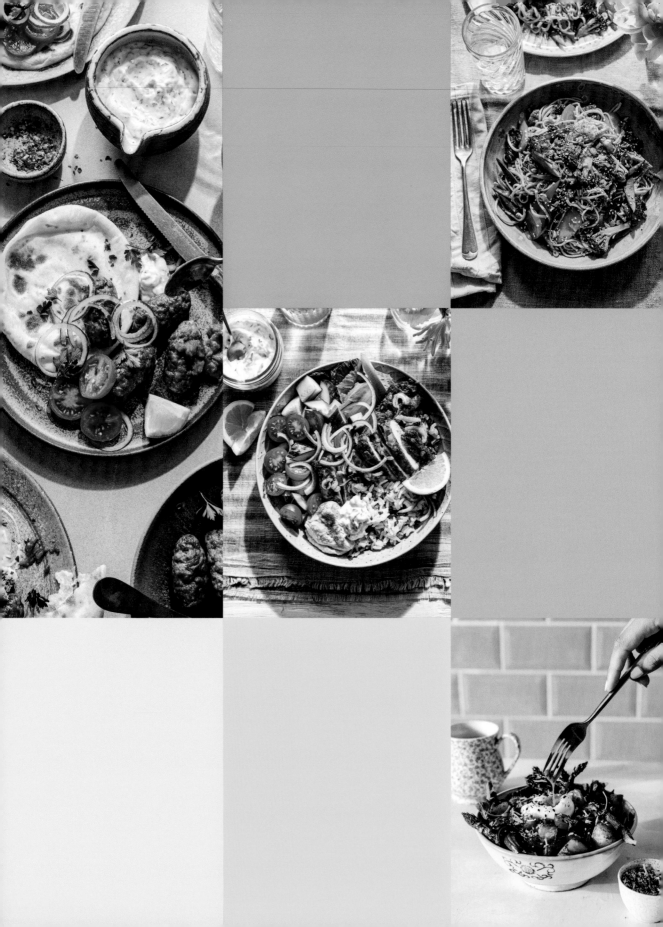

Slimming
EATS

Healthy, delicious recipes – 100+ under 500 calories

Siobhan Wightman

Photography by Haarala Hamilton

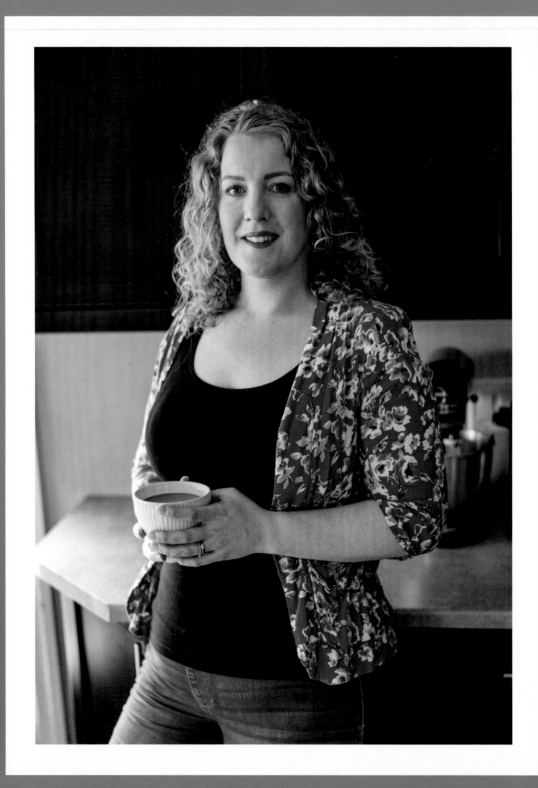

Introduction

Hello and welcome to my debut cookbook! I'm Siobhan, the founder of Slimming Eats, a blog I created back in 2009 as a place to record my own weight-loss journey and share what I was cooking in the process. I never for one minute imagined what it would become. For me, it was just a visual diary of my journey, an outlet to keep me accountable and document my recipes as I went along – but gradually people started to comment on my posts, and then leave messages saying they had made one of my recipes and loved it, or they would share how much weight they had lost using them.

Over the years the blog has empowered so many people to take control of their weight loss and healthy living lifestyle, and it has become an inspiring community. The support has been amazing, and in turn, the Slimming Eats community has helped me stay motivated through the ups and downs of life. Fast-forward to where we're at now: over 8 million people visited the Slimming Eats website in 2020 and as of summer 2021, I have 1.5 million followers across my socials, which still completely astounds me!

It has definitely become a full-time job – I don't have a team of people working behind the scenes – and it is very busy, but it brings me a huge amount of happiness each day. I develop, test, cook, edit and photograph every single one of the recipes on my website and the technical stuff is managed by my amazing husband, Gavin – without him and his knowledge I think it would have become too much a long time ago.

As well as creating all the content I run my Facebook group, where I give my readers tips, encouragement and advice. I love the friendly, supportive environment it has become, and the fact that members have been able to get to know me, not just some faceless person behind the scenes; they understand all the thought and process that goes into all my creations and I can't thank them enough for the fantastic support they give me in return. It's so rewarding to watch the progress my readers make from following my recipes, and to see the pictures they share of the dishes they cook from Slimming Eats.

I had originally wanted to keep my website as the only source of my recipes and accessible to everyone. Truthfully, I am a bit of an introvert, and I'm quite shy too, so putting myself out there on social media can sometimes have its downsides. It is one of the main reasons I have declined doing a cookbook for so long, and let me tell you I've turned down many offers. Then along came the lovely Lauren at Yellow Kite and she didn't give up on me, constantly checking in, but not harassing me and hoping I'd change my mind. After years of my readers begging me to write a book every day, and with almost 1,000 recipes available on my website, I began to feel that now is the right time, so I said, 'OK, let's do it'!

My family and friends are huge supporters of what I do and my children's biggest dream, or so they keep telling me, is to see Mummy's cookbook on the shelf at the bookshop, so I couldn't let them down. So by request, here it is. I have crafted 100 new recipes, and I've also included a selection of my most loved favourites from the website, so there is something for everyone, old fans and new.

I hope you enjoy using it as much as I have enjoyed creating it. It has been a labour of love, but a lot of fun – much of the food in these pages is inspired by dishes I have enjoyed locally, and by the fail-safe meals I have cooked for my family, as well as taking inspiration from my readers by looking at what they cook most from the blog.

I have crafted 100 new recipes, and I've also included a selection of my most loved favourites from the website, so there really is something for everyone

A Love for Cooking Real Food

I don't call myself an experienced chef by any means, I'm just a home cook who loves experimenting with ingredients and flavours. I'm not trained professionally, so I still find it rather surreal that so many people tell me how much they love my recipes. I take inspiration from the countries I've visited and lived in. I was born in London, but I've lived in Ireland, Kent, the Midlands and now Canada, and being close to the US gives me great travel opportunities. I also became accustomed to different cuisines from a very young age because of my dad's occupation, which was working with ventilation in restaurants and takeaways, along with designing and building wok cookers used in Chinese cuisine. He used to drag me to jobs with him and I could see dishes being made in the kitchens. You will find these influences in the recipes on my website and in this book, with Chinese-, Indian-, Mexican- and Thai-inspired recipes, to name just a few.

My passion for cooking comes from seeing my mother cook from scratch and learning basic skills from her. She always managed to make a delicious meal from even the most basic of ingredients, nothing posh or fancy, with no measuring whatsoever... just real home-cooked food. I think the fact she was Irish meant she learnt how not to waste ingredients from a young age. It's probably why now, as a mum myself, I am so focused on healthy home-cooked food that the whole family can enjoy. I don't want to cook separate meals, so it's important that my children will eat my recipes too, which is why I am so set on using natural ingredients as much as I can and limiting all those artificial ingredients and 'diet foods'.

My background has always been in the creative field. I studied and received a degree in fine art, and have been creating or making things from a very young age, so when it comes to food, I guess my creative side comes out there too. When I went to university, I began to cook for myself and I often craved and cooked hearty meals (as well as eating the typical student food like beans on toast). The kitchen became my happy place and I relished the challenge of combining whatever ingredients I have available into a healthy, hearty meal. Of course there are occasions when things don't turn out how I expect them to, but that's all part of the fun of it and I don't give up easily, sticking with the recipe until it's just perfect and passes the taste test from the family.

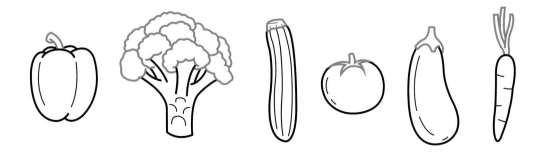

My Weight-loss Journey

I can't pinpoint exactly when I started gaining weight, but it was some time in my late teens, when events in my life caused depression and anxiety and led to unhealthy eating habits. I probably tried every diet out there, but they were never maintainable long-term, not least because the food was just boring and uninspiring, as most diet recipes are. My weight was like a yo-yo, up and down, up and down, and each time I came off a restrictive diet I would gain even more weight than when I started. It wasn't ever a healthy approach, losing weight fast then reverting back to my original eating habits, and we all know it doesn't work.

My weight gain got to an all-time high after the birth of my son. First came the misconception that you can eat what you like when pregnant, and I definitely did that, resulting in huge weight gain, which in turn caused lots of health issues in my pregnancy. And on top of that there was the very traumatic birth. I didn't really know it at the time, but I was suffering with PTSD (Post Traumatic Stress Disorder) after my son's birth – I rarely left the house and ate myself into oblivion, gaining even more weight. I just focused on caring for my son, who I loved more than anything in the world, and stopped looking after myself. I was a mum and nothing else. I didn't realize or care that being a mum also meant looking after myself.

Just when I felt I was regaining control again and had managed to lose a bit of weight with yet another restrictive diet, my family took on a massive life change by moving to Canada. But just like before, the stress and anxiety of such a big move led to yet more comfort eating and weight gain, especially with all the new cuisines and food at our disposal. It was like being on a permanent holiday, until I caught a glimpse of myself in a photograph that my husband had taken of me holding my son. I was so unhappy at what I saw that I knew I had to make changes to my lifestyle, and those changes needed to be for good. No more restrictive diets or short-term fixes... and that resulted in the creation of Slimming Eats, and with that the loss of over 60lbs.

This time my approach was different: I stopped relying on convenient comfort foods in packages and restricting myself, and instead went back to creating and cooking the foods I loved, in my own home, from scratch, using healthy, fresh ingredients (just like my mother had done). I soon realized that I didn't need to eat boring restrictive meals to lose weight, that with just a few changes and tweaks to cut the calories I could have all the delicious meals that I loved.

But as with all things in life, it's never a clear-cut journey when it comes to weight loss.

When we finally decided to extend our family, I was faced with infertility issues due to PCOS (Polycystic Ovary Syndrome) and again more stress. But unlike before, where I would have just piled on the weight, this time I took control and things were different. Eventually, by sticking to a balanced healthy eating plan and having an amazing and understanding doctor on board who helped with my PCOS and the infertility side of things, I finally became pregnant with my daughter. And unlike in my first pregnancy, where I gained far too much weight, this time I gained hardly any and I felt fantastic. The pregnancy was healthy and I had no complications at all, and even more surprising, I was back in my pre-pregnancy clothes just a week after giving birth.

Several years later, getting older and living in a different country away from family has brought its own challenges. My journey has not always been straightforward and easy, and there are times when I've struggled. Being in another country when parents begin to get older and ill is not something that can be fully appreciated when deciding that emigration might be a fun adventure. Being an only child, living far away and seeing my mum slowly declining through dementia, brought on a whole heap of worry, anxiety and stress, which in turn took its toll on my mental health. As you can imagine, my healthy eating then took a backseat. Then a few years later came the added upset and stress of finally losing my mum to the dementia. Losing weight, even with healthy eating, was not as easy as before, and it can sometimes be hard to stay motivated when you are working hard but not seeing results. Finally I was diagnosed with hypothyroidism and an autoimmune disease in 2020, and I am still struggling with the symptoms – I have to be extra vigilant about weight gain, as getting back to a healthy weight and staying there is so much more difficult for me than it was a decade ago.

The important part is to own your weight-loss journey. There will be ups and downs along the way, good days and bad days, but the main thing is to do what is comfortable for you and what makes you happy and is sustainable. The road isn't always easy and simple, sometimes it'll be rocky, but if you start building positive habits and really fall in love with cooking proper meals and using real ingredients, this is an excellent grounding to fall back on, even when you take a few steps back. Try not to deprive yourself of the things you love the most – remember, moderation is key.

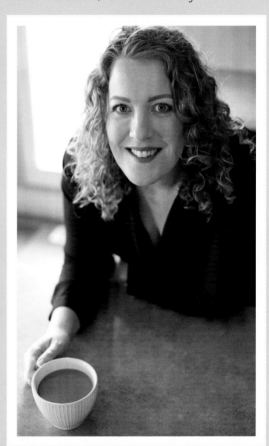

Useful Kitchen Equipment

These are my must-have Slimming Eats kitchen items that will set you up for your journey ahead and help make prepping and cooking that little bit easier.

UTENSILS

Having a variety of different utensils is important – as well as the specific ones listed below, wooden or silicone spatulas/spoons (especially if using non-stick cookware, as you don't want to scratch the coating), vegetable peelers, julienne peelers, graters, zesters, whisks and kitchen scissors (great for removing fat and skin from meat) are all handy to have.

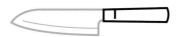

KNIFE AND SHARPENING BLOCK

A good-quality knife for chopping and slicing is essential, and I can't recommend Santoku knives enough. They originated in Japan and are very popular. I own several, and I love them so much. The blade is slightly curved, so it can rock on the board for easy dicing and chopping. Always make sure you keep the blade of your knife sharp to ensure precise chopping and no mishaps. Most kitchen mishaps with knives are caused by using a blunt knife.

KITCHEN SCALES

For low-calorie cooking and baking, these are a must, as ingredients often need to be precise to ensure you are sticking to your calorie goal. It's far too easy to underestimate if you are just guessing. You don't need expensive ones, but I do recommend digital.

MEASURING CUPS AND SPOONS

These are very popular measuring tools in North America and are becoming common in the UK now, even though the UK is on the metric system. It's because of their ease of use for measuring things. I converted to these quickly when I moved to Canada, and you will see me use them a lot on the blog.

GOOD-QUALITY NON-STICK FRYING PANS (SKILLET) AND SAUCEPANS

Perfect for low-calorie cooking and for using smaller amounts of oil. Overall I prefer ceramic-coated non-stick cookware.

CAST IRON PAN

I love my seasoned cast iron cookware – it's perfect for searing meats like chicken, steak, etc. and will last you a lifetime if you care for it properly.

CASSEROLE/DUTCH OVEN

As I mentioned, I like cast iron cookware. Most brands come with a lifetime warranty, and I recommend the enamelled brands like Le Creuset, though there are cheaper alternatives available too. These are wonderful for casseroles and stews, as they can be transferred from stovetop to oven.

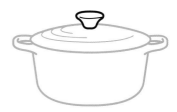

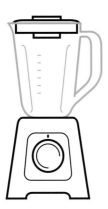

BLENDER

A definite must-have. I use mine so much that it lives on my kitchen counter. They are essential for soups, sauces and anything that needs blending. You don't need to spend a fortune on a counter-top one if you are on a budget – the hand-held stick immersion blenders will also do the job.

FOOD PROCESSOR

Some blenders have a food processor bowl attachment, so if you are limited on space, this might be the option for you. Mini food processors are great for making curry pastes, hummus, etc. when you don't need the large bowl of a big food processor.

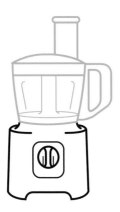

PRESSURE COOKER

This is not needed for any of the recipes in the book, but it's probably one of my most used appliances after my stove, and it's perfect for anyone who has a busy schedule. I use mine for all sorts – making yoghurt, curries, soups, casseroles, pasta dishes, rice dishes, homemade broth, etc. You can even cook a whole chicken in a pressure cooker.

SLOW COOKER

Slow cookers are magic for when you want to get a dish started in the morning and have it ready for dinner time. Most electric pressure cookers have a slow cooker option, so if you are looking to add one of those to your collection of gadgets, you may not need a slow cooker as well.

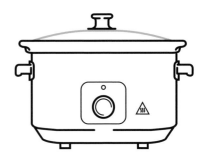

AIR FRYER

While not needed for the recipes in this book, this is an amazing gadget, and there are so many options available compared to a few years ago. You can get ones with a paddle that will rotate the food for you, or ones with a basket – either works well, so go for what you can afford. Air fryers work well for foods that are usually deep-fried because they use much less oil – usually just a tablespoon, if that.

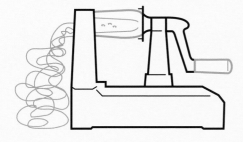

VEGETABLE SPIRALIZER

There are so many different types of spiralizer available. You can even get an attachment for the KitchenAid mixer, if you are lucky enough to own one of those. A spiralizer is a handy gadget for making low-calorie sides for your main course. I recommend a counter-top one rather than hand-held, because the counter-top ones generally come with four or more blades and can spiralize all kinds of vegetables, whereas the hand-held ones can generally only spiralize stick-shaped vegetables. I use mine a lot, and it's a simple way to incorporate vegetables into the plates of fussy eaters. Vegetables I like to spiralize are courgettes (zucchini), carrots, butternut squash, sweet potatoes, parsnips, turnips, swede, celeriac (celery root) – pretty much any hard veg will spiral and you can even do some fruits and things like cucumber. You can easily reduce the calories in dishes by using only half the required pasta and replacing the rest with spiralized veg.

VEGETABLE CHOPPER

This is not an essential gadget, but if you struggle with good knife skills or don't feel confident using a knife for chopping and dicing, it's a good option to have. Like the spiralizer, it also usually comes with a few different blade sizes for chopping veg small or large.

BAKING TRAYS/DISHES

I cook a lot of traybakes for my family, so I like to have a good selection of different-sized baking trays. My favourites are aluminium baking trays (Nordicware), as they come in various sizes including an extra large. Some baking dishes in assorted sizes are useful too – large ones for things like pasta bakes and small ones for single serve, desserts, baked oats, etc..

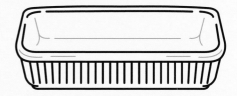

PARCHMENT PAPER

Unbleached parchment paper is something I use a lot. It will protect your baking trays and stop food sticking, meaning less clean-up afterwards – and as a busy mum, I am all for that.

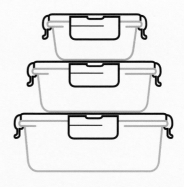

FOOD CONTAINERS

I love batch cooking or making extra when I cook, so food containers are a must. I've recently ditched plastic, though, and changed to glass containers. Most can go straight into the oven, meaning you don't need to transfer food from one container to another when you want to reheat it, and even better, there's less washing up.

Store Cupboard Essentials

BUILDING UP YOUR STORE CUPBOARD/PANTRY

When you first begin cooking your own food in an attempt to be healthier, it can become overwhelming, looking at all the store cupboard ingredients, spices, and so on. My main tip is to take it one week at a time – don't try to buy everything at once, as it will become much too costly and is unnecessary. Instead plan your week's meals and buy only the ingredients you need, gradually building up your collection of spices and store cupboard ingredients as you go along.

SHOPPING ON A BUDGET

When planning meals, I try to keep to a healthy balance of fresh ingredients, but also to have the occasional meal that uses dried pulses, grains, legumes, pasta, etc., which tends to be more budget-friendly. You certainly don't want to be eating expensive cuts of steak every night if money is tight. Balance is key.

For dry ingredients, shop in bulk where you can, as it usually works out much cheaper, especially for rice, lentils, beans, etc. Tinned are a great option too, but these can sometimes be high in sodium. So overall, I prefer to buy dried for things like lentils, beans and pulses.

While fresh vegetables and fruits are always my preferred choice, a selection of frozen fruit and vegetables is always good to have on hand and is great for those on a budget, though not always possible if you don't have a big freezer space.

If you are lucky enough to have a market nearby, you'll be able to pick up fruit and vegetables at a cheaper price than in the supermarkets, and some butchers will do family packs of different meats.

SOURCING HARD-TO-FIND INGREDIENTS

There are very few recipes in the book that use hard-to-find ingredients, but occasionally in an ingredients list there may be an item you haven't heard of before, usually in cuisines from around the world that need a certain ingredient for that authentic taste. I will always try to suggest a swap if I can, but sometimes it's just not possible.

My best advice is to look for Chinese or Indian grocers in your area, as they are excellent for stocking special ingredients. European and Caribbean markets are good too, and in some cities there may be world markets, which hold products from all over the world. Some larger supermarkets have international aisles, and it's worth checking those out, and of course, last but not least, there is always online. You can find pretty much anything on websites such as Amazon.

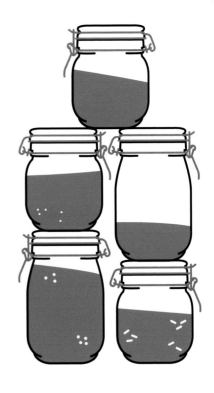

STORE CUPBOARD INGREDIENTS

Having a stocked store cupboard will help you pull together delicious meals easily, affordably and healthily. These are my store cupboard essentials.

Rice
(long-grain, brown, arborio, jasmine)

Pasta
(various shapes – penne, spaghetti, lasagne sheets)

Couscous

Quinoa

Wholegrains
(pearl barley, bulgur wheat)

Oats
(both rolled and steel cut)

Dried lentils
(brown, green and red)

Dried beans
(chickpeas, kidney beans and haricot beans are cheap to buy in bulk and will last ages)

Tinned beans and lentils
(great for quick meals)

Tinned fish
(tuna, salmon and sardines are great for creating budget-friendly meals for the family)

Cooking oils
(olive oil, avocado oil, ghee, coconut oil)

Spray oil
(I pick 100% oil varieties, no preservatives, fillers or propellants)

Sesame oil
(this is more for flavour than cooking with but important for Chinese dishes)

Stock
(I prefer fat-free broth in cartons, but stock cubes are fine too)

Soy sauce
(tamari for gluten-free or coconut aminos for soy-free)

Sauces
(oyster sauce, black bean sauce, hoisin sauce, fish sauce)

Tinned coconut milk
(light and regular)

Mirin

Shaoxing wine

Sriracha sauce

Worcestershire sauce

Tabasco

Vinegars
(white wine, red wine, rice, balsamic)

Sweeteners
(brown sugar, maple syrup, honey, granulated sweetener – I use erythritol)

Passata

Tinned chopped tomatoes

Tomato purée (paste)

Plain (all-purpose) flour

Cornflour (cornstarch), arrowroot or tapioca flour
(all good for thickening sauces)

Baking powder

Bicarbonate of soda (baking soda)

Extracts
(vanilla and almond)

There are far too many for me to actually list them all, oh my I have built up a quite a collection. My advice would be to start with the basics and each week or fortnight buy a new one until you build up a good selection. Spices are the element that adds all that lovely flavour to your food.

Here are the basics I really do recommend getting. Start off with these and go from there. You can gradually add to those as you start cooking my recipes:	Then a more extensive list of spices I like to have on hand are:
Salt	Dried herbs (oregano, basil, thyme, rosemary, mint, parsley)
Black pepper	Cayenne pepper
Mixed (Italian) herbs	Garam masala
Cinnamon	Turmeric
Garlic powder	Smoked paprika
Onion powder	Sumac
Ground cumin	Cumin seeds
Ground coriander	Mustard powder
Chilli powder (mild and hot – I like Kashmiri for curries)	Ginger
Curry powder	Cloves
Paprika	Green cardamom pods
	Cinnamon bark
	Bay leaves

Slimming Eats Style

Cooking Tips and Notes

LEAN MEATS

To reduce calories in a dish I will always trim any visible fat from meat, even if it says 'lean' or 'extra lean' on the packaging. Even boneless and skinless chicken thighs can often have quite a bit of fat still attached. I use kitchen scissors for this.

However, that said, if you want a little bit of skin from a roast chicken or the crispy fat on a piece of bacon, have it and count it. Remember not to deprive yourself too much of the things you like, as that is not maintainable – everything is fine in moderation.

For minced (ground) meat I try to keep to 5% fat. I don't generally like to go lower than this if it's for burgers, meatballs, etc., as the meat can become a bit dry if it's too lean.

For stews and casserole type dishes where chicken is the main protein, I always use thighs, never breast. I find thighs stay tender in these recipes and add flavour to the dish overall. Chicken breast doesn't take long to cook, so can quickly become overcooked.

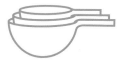

MEASUREMENT OF INGREDIENTS

You will notice that I sometimes give precise measurements for things like onions and carrots. Stating just 1 onion or 1 carrot is fine in some cases, but as these differ in size there are occasions where the amount needs to be given more precisely.

Make sure when it comes to things like tablespoons and teaspoons that you are using accurate measuring spoons and levelling off (never use heaped). I don't recommend using normal cutlery for a tablespoon or a teaspoon, because these can really vary in size.

OIL SPRAYS

I believe in using real ingredients, so if I feel a recipe needs a little bit of olive oil or similar I will use it. 1 or 2 tablespoons in a meal for 4 is not going to be much calorie-wise.

I do use oil sprays, but only when I feel it won't affect the overall taste of the dish. Sometimes you just won't get the same flavour using these. The oil sprays that I prefer to use are ones that don't contain emulsifiers, and where the ingredients are just oil, but that is a personal preference, so use the type you prefer or whatever is available.

For cooking fats, my favourites are olive oil, real butter, ghee (amazing for Indian-style dishes), avocado oil and coconut oil. The last three have high smoke points so are great options to use. Don't be scared to use real ingredients when you're on your weight-loss journey. Losing weight doesn't mean resorting to 'diet foods' – just use them sparingly instead.

STOCK

Where you see stock mentioned in a recipe, there are a couple of things to note. I generally like to buy cartons of fat-free stock or make my own. These just have much cleaner ingredients and taste fresher. Occasionally in an emergency, if I don't have those on hand, I will use bouillon or stock cubes, and there are a few things to note if these are your preferred choice.

Different stock cubes require different amounts of liquid. For example, some stock cubes are mixed with just 180ml (6fl oz) of water for 180ml of stock, while others you mix with a lot more water – you need to check the label and ensure you use the correct amount, otherwise your stock could be too weak in flavour or too salty, neither desirable outcomes!

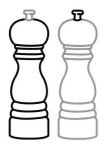

SALT AND PEPPER

Seasoning with salt and pepper is always to an acquired taste and is a must with any savoury recipe, so my measures are usually just a guideline. These are basic flavour enhancers, so get into the habit of tasting as you cook, adjusting the seasoning as needed and using your instinct. Far too often we think that to add flavour we need to add a whole load of different spices, when the majority of the time all that is needed is a little extra salt and pepper. Those who are used to a low-sodium diet may wish to use far less than someone who likes a lot of flavour, so this is why it's important to adjust the amount to your own taste – it's one of the reasons you always see salt and pepper on a table.

ADJUSTING SEASONINGS

Don't be scared of adjusting seasonings to your own taste too – if you don't like food too spicy, add a smaller amount, or if there is a seasoning you don't like, as long as it's not a major part of the recipe ingredients, it should be fine to omit or swap it with something else. As you begin to cook more and more meals from scratch, you will get used to knowing which seasonings pair well with things.

GRANULATED SWEETENERS

There are so many different types of sweeteners out there that it can be hard to know which one is best to use and, importantly, not all sweeteners are created equal.

Generally, I prefer to use real, natural sweeteners like maple syrup or honey. But sometimes, where I want to keep the calories low and where it doesn't affect the overall taste of the recipe, you'll see a recipe mention granulated sweetener, and this will always be a naturally derived sweetener called erythritol. There are lots of different brands of this type of sweetener out there, but most of the time it is used in the exact same quantity as you would use sugar, and it tastes very close to the real thing too, which is why it's my preferred choice.

Other sweeteners may have an overpowering aftertaste or may require you to use more or a lot less, so always check the packaging if you choose to use a different one. Otherwise it could affect the taste or bake.

THICKENING SAUCES

Like a thicker sauce or gravy? There are various ways to thicken a sauce – the easiest low-calorie way is to use vegetables as a base and blend them like a soup. This is perfect for fussy eaters and will add flavour, thickness and depth to a sauce. But sometimes we don't have time for that, so a quicker way is to use a little bit of starch such as cornflour (cornstarch), arrowroot or tapioca. The great thing about these is that most of them are gluten-free and you don't need to cook them with butter to make a roux, which is perfect when you're trying to save calories. To use as a thickener, I generally use 1 tablespoon per 240ml (1 cup) of liquid (occasionally, depending on the other ingredients, you may need more or less), but don't add it straight into your sauce or it will go lumpy – mix it with a little cold water to make a slurry and then you can stir it into the sauce and gently heat until thickened.

OVEN TEMPERATURES

All the recipes on Slimming Eats use a regular non-fan oven. Fan oven temperatures, however, are included in the book – these are usually 20°C (68°F) lower than a regular oven temperature. But I always recommend getting to know your own oven, as some may need to go even lower. Various things can affect how an oven bakes, like high and low altitudes, and in older fan ovens the temperature may not be even.

STOVETOP TEMPERATURES

Sauces not reducing or thickening? The biggest culprit for this is that the heat is too low. Even when simmering, a sauce should still be bubbling – if it isn't bubbling at all, that sauce isn't going anywhere. So make sure you don't have the heat too low. At the same time, you don't want to try to speed up cooking by having the heat too high, as then you risk burning and ruining the food completely. It's a fine balance!

For frying/searing you want a medium–high heat generally, which is enough to give a nice searing or browning but not so high that the food cooks too fast and burns.

For boiling, where there is a lot of liquid (for example soups and stews), you can turn the heat right up to the highest setting – you want to see vigorous bubbles in the liquid, which happens when the temperature gets to around 100°C (212°F).

For simmering you can turn the heat down to around medium for sauces (rapid simmer), or medium–low to give a gentle simmer for soups and stews.

SAUTÉEING/BROWNING/ROASTING

When it comes to browning ingredients, make sure you don't rush this. It's the vital step that adds flavour to a dish – if you rush it will likely burn, and if you don't brown the ingredient enough, your entire dish could end up looking a bit pale and lacking in flavour. Take the time to get that lovely sear on the meat, which may mean browning it in two batches if your pan is small (and never overcrowd a pan for this vital step).

This also applies for roasting/baking – use a baking tray or dish that is big enough for all the ingredients in an even layer. If they are piled up or too close together, this can result in them steaming when ideally you want heat to penetrate around all the ingredients.

You will also see me use stock occasionally as a way to really soften down vegetables instead of using oil, a great trick for low-fat cooking that I learnt many years ago. Instead of using heaps of oil to sauté or brown, you just add a little bit of stock and reduce it down around the vegetables, then keep adding more stock a little at a time until the veggies are lovely and golden and softened. It's kind of the same process as making risotto, and it works really well for adding flavour as a base to so many recipes.

To Freeze or Not to Freeze?

TO FREEZE OR NOT TO FREEZE?

The recipes that are suitable for freezing in the book will have this freezer icon next to them:

I have given the freezer-friendly icon only to the recipes that I am happy to freeze, but there may be some dishes without the icon that you might like to freeze too.

Slimming Eats strongly believes in creating healthy meals that the whole family can enjoy, which is why most of the recipes in this book serve 4, because my family consists of 4: me, my husband and my two children. But one of the most frequent questions I get is: can this be frozen? Especially if someone is cooking a recipe that serves 4 but is making it for 2 or even 1. The short answer is that really there isn't much you can't freeze. However, it comes down to personal preference as to whether you like a reheated meal out of the freezer.

PASTA

Many people don't care for reheated pasta, because it can become soft and overcooked. But that doesn't mean you can't freeze pasta dishes, you totally can – again, it's a personal preference. With pasta bakes the best results are often achieved by freezing ahead of the final cooking step – so if you are cooking a bigger portion than you need, before baking I'd portion into 2 dishes and freeze one, bake the other.

DISHES WITH NO SAUCE

Dishes with minimal sauce are sometimes not favourable for freezing because they can become a little dry when reheated, especially if the dish contains lean meat such as chicken breast or pork.

RICE DISHES

There is often a debate about this, but cooked rice is actually safe to reheat or freeze, as long as you follow these guidelines. You must ensure you refrigerate or freeze the rice quickly (as soon as it's cooled down) – don't leave it at room temperature for any length of time. It can be reheated once only, and make sure it's piping hot all the way through.

SOUPS

Soups are great for freezing. However, soups that contain rice and pasta can end up with very little broth when reheated, or the pasta can be overcooked and mushy (check out defrosting tips on the opposite page).

EGGS

Eggs can sometimes have a weird rubbery texture when frozen and reheated, which is mainly because they've become overcooked. A few exceptions are crustless quiches/frittatas, which tend to freeze OK, and the eggs inside the Make-ahead Sausage, Egg and Cheese English Muffins on page 38 (because the egg is sandwiched between other items, it freezes and reheats perfectly).

GARLIC AND GINGER

With garlic, it's useful to freeze whole bulbs, so you can just pop out a clove as you need it for a recipe. And you can freeze whole peeled roots of fresh ginger, and just grate them from frozen.

DEFROSTING AND REHEATING

While some meals can be reheated from frozen, for best results I personally prefer to defrost in the fridge and then reheat once defrosted.

Things like soups can be reheated on the stovetop or in the microwave.

Pasta bakes, potato-topped pies – you can reheat these in the oven or microwave.

Always ensure that any food you reheat is piping hot throughout.

If you do choose to freeze soups that contain pasta or rice, here are a couple of tips: either freeze portions without the rice/pasta and then just add cooked rice or pasta when you reheat, or add some additional stock to the soup before reheating.

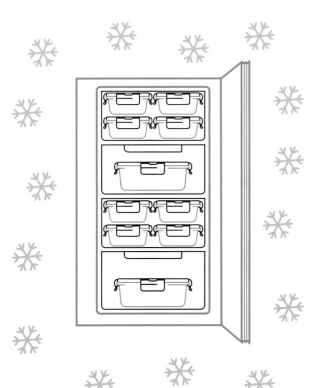

A NOTE ON CONTAINERS FOR FREEZING

There are various different types of containers available for freezing food, including bags and meal prep containers. I freeze meals in glass freezer-friendly containers. If you make sure they are oven safe, you can then defrost and reheat in the same container, which comes in really handy.

Using containers that are all the same shape can be space-saving – plus if you opt for square or rectangular tubs you can stack them right up to the corners of your freezer drawer and not waste valuable space – especially useful if you have limited freezer availability.

I stopped using labels to label my tubs – why? Most of them fall off and then I have no idea what is in the actual container or when it was frozen. I can't remember the number of times I have had what I call a 'freezer surprise', which is a tub you remove from the freezer and have no idea what it actually contains until you defrost and reheat it, because the labels are nowhere to be seen. Instead I use markers and write directly on the container, which is another nice thing about glass containers – the marker is easy to clean off.

Make sure you clearly note what is in the container (some people like to include the calories, etc.) and always put the date of freezing – that way you can see what needs to be used up first. Most cooked food that is frozen is best used within 3 months.

If you are freezing things like burgers/pancakes/cakes, etc. in one container, I always recommend adding a sheet of waxed paper between each individual one. This will ensure they are easy to take apart if you only want to remove one or two at a time.

It's easier if you freeze in portions rather than one big container, as that way no food is wasted, especially if you only actually want one serving. However, if you have a big family you may find it easier to freeze in one container.

Some Final Important Bits!

NOTES ON DIETARY TAGS AND NUTRITIONAL ANALYSIS

V	VEGETARIAN
DF	DAIRY-FREE
GF	GLUTEN-FREE
	FREEZER-FRIENDLY

Beside each recipe you will see these symbols, which state which recipes are vegetarian, dairy-free and gluten-free, plus which are freezer-friendly.

Each recipe also features a full nutritional analysis. This is per portion, and has been made with the following ingredients (unless otherwise stated): skimmed milk, wholemeal (whole wheat) low-calorie bread, skinless and lean meat, fat-free yoghurt, granulated sweetener and light cream cheese. They exclude optional items and 'to serve' items, so bear this in mind if you're adding in optional extras.

When a recipe includes the freezer icon, it can be frozen and stored in the freezer for a maximum of 3 months.

LOW-CARB SIDES

If you are trying to keep the calories low in a meal, there are some great low-carb options in the sides chapter (page 232) and on the website.

One of my favourite low-carb vegetables is cauliflower, mainly because it is such a versatile ingredient. You can roast it, steam it, stir-fry it, and turn it into rice or even mash.

SWAPPING INGREDIENTS

Don't be afraid to swap certain vegetables and other ingredients for ones you prefer if there is something you don't like. So long as you keep to around the same quantity and the cooking time is about the same, it should work fine. If your swap needs more cooking, or less, you will need to adjust the recipe to account for that.

Sometimes, however, especially when following a recipe for the first time, it's best to keep to it as precisely as possible, so that you will be more aware of timings and what you can and can't swap when you make it the second time.

GLUTEN-FREE, DAIRY-FREE AND VEGETARIAN

If a swap can be made to make a recipe suitable for those with certain allergies or dietary restrictions, you will see a suggestion underneath the recipe. If you're swapping in dairy-free and gluten-free alternatives, please note these will alter the nutritional analysis.

Of course these are just suggestions, so check that the alternative products or ingredients you use in any recipes from Slimming Eats are free from allergens (gluten-free, egg-free, soy-free and/ or dairy-free, for example).

My recipes all use gluten-free and dairy-free stock, condiments and spice mixes, but always check the labels to ensure the products you wish to use are gluten-free and dairy-free. If you or someone you're cooking for has dietary requirements, be sure to especially check the labels for condiments and stock.

I've done rounds of gluten-free and dairy-free in the past for health reasons, and there are great gluten-free and dairy-free products that I still use.

For pasta: my favourite gluten-free option is brown rice pasta, but there are lots of others out there too, made from corn, quinoa, and even lentils and beans.

For milks: cashew milk is my favourite non-dairy milk – it doesn't have a strong nutty flavour and is lovely and creamy, plus, as a big tea drinker, it's the only milk I have found that works against the tannin in tea without separating.

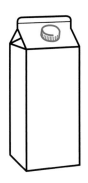

GETTING YOUR 5-A-DAY – VEGGIES COME FIRST

My biggest tip for ensuring you get a good balance of vegetables on your plate is to think about vegetables first.

For example, when cooking, instead of thinking of the protein first and what you can serve with it, look at what vegetables you have. It's much easier to include more vegetables on your plate if you think this way. Sometimes it won't be possible, like just before a grocery shop, but it really does help me keep my meals well-balanced and stops me finding vegetables that have spoiled in the vegetable drawer of my fridge. I hate food waste! (By the way, a hack for keeping that unused half of an avocado fresh is to leave the stone in and wrap it in foil – it will keep for a few days in the fridge.)

Try to source unusual fruits and vegetables you haven't tried before – it makes food more interesting. I am lucky that where I live we have so many different types of fruits and vegetables available to us – some I had never seen until I moved to Canada – and it makes eating healthily so much more enjoyable and varied.

Most vegetables are low in calories, so they are the perfect food for bulking out your plate to make a meal more filling. This means you can enjoy a small serving of the foods you love, but still keep yourself satisfied by filling yourself up with vegetables.

VEGETARIAN SWAPS

I have included notes on how to make specific dishes vegetarian on the recipe pages, but if you fancy trying to make something vegetarian yourself, here are my favourite vegetarian alternatives to meat.

Aubergine (eggplant)
(when roasted, aubergines have an umami flavour and a meaty feel)

Balsamic tomatoes
(for a sweet, salty and flavourful addition or salad topper – page 45)

Beans
(chickpeas, kidney beans and haricot beans are brilliant for adding extra protein and texture)

Butternut squash cubes or sweet potato chunks
(for a nutty, caramelized flavour)

Cauliflower
(sprinkled with herbs and spices, cauliflower can be transformed into the star of any dish)

Leafy greens
(spinach and kale are great for adding extra nutrients into omelettes and stews)

Lentils
(these work nicely as a mince substitute)

Meat substitutes
(tofu, seitan, tempeh and soya pieces are full of protein and have similar textures to meat)

Mushrooms
(grilled portobello mushrooms are great burger patty alternatives and oyster, porcini and button mushrooms are wonderful meat substitutes in stews, casseroles, pasta dishes and soups)

Paneer
(this is an Indian cheese that can be used in stir-fries and curries to add a creamy, chewy texture)

Peppers
(raw, roasted or sautéed – perfect for adding crunch or soft sweetness)

STAYING MOTIVATED

When it comes to healthy eating, losing motivation is one of the most common causes of falling off the wagon, and the biggest culprits are not enjoying your food or depriving yourself too much – as mentioned before, I've been there... This was one of the main reasons I started Slimming Eats. I found all the low-calorie recipes that were available just so bland and boring, and not like the delicious home-cooked foods I was used to.

It's one of the reasons I believe in using real ingredients, instead of lots of low-fat, sugar-free, diet products. If you only keep to those, you will quickly become bored and uninspired. With this book, you will be able to eat proper, tasty food while still remaining healthy. All those calorific ingredients you think you should be avoiding don't actually need to be avoided at all – it's just a question of using those ingredients in sensible amounts. Switching your style of cooking to a healthier alternative will also reduce calories. An example of this would be air-frying/baking instead of deep-frying.

If you struggle to put meal ideas together at the drop of a hat, meal planning is definitely advised. There is nothing worse than coming home from a long day at work hungry and not having anything planned, as we all know the likely scenario here. Those are the times you are going to grab something unhealthy, and it probably won't satisfy you either, and quick fixes always lead to grabbing even more unhealthy stuff later. Meal prep is useful if you work a really busy schedule. Set aside a free day each week when you can cook a few meals in advance to have on hand for those busy days.

That aside, I know all too well that there are various things in life that can affect motivation: illness, depression, weight not coming off as fast as we'd like, chaotic schedules, coming back from holiday, the list goes on. So just take your journey one day at a time – it's not a race, it's a lifestyle change. You will have bad days, because that's life. The key is not to let one bad day undo all the good days and become weeks or months of bad days.

Which goes back to what I said before, about not depriving yourself so much that it feels like a diet. Restrictive diets are not maintainable and they make you unhappy.

For helping with motivation, one of the things I suggest is taking up a non-food hobby that will fill those moments when you are likely to want to grab food out of boredom. It can be anything you like, but activities that keep the mind busy and occupied are a great choice. I like to draw and paint or work on my family tree. But when it's warm outside I also like to get the family out for a walk at a local nature park, as I love seeing local wildlife.

Joining online support groups is another option, you can meet others on a similar journey to yourself and motivate each other. Facebook groups (Slimming Eats has its own little support group on Facebook) and Instagram are inspiring places for this.

Keeping a food diary, where you can record your meals and weight losses, is another handy idea. You can look back on what you ate when you had a really good week, or see what you can improve on with the not so good weeks. But don't expect huge losses every week. There will be weeks where you have small weight losses, stay the same and sometimes make small gains.

Exercise is another key factor. However, it may not be possible for everyone on a healthy eating journey, because sometimes illness or work can get in the way. With an autoimmune disease which sometimes leaves me so fatigued that I struggle to get out of bed some mornings, I know that what comes easy to some is not so easy for others. However, when I do include some exercise in my week I feel much better for it, which means I feel much more motivated too. It doesn't need to be anything extreme – just reaching a daily step goal using a fitness watch can be a fruitful win and finding a type of exercise you enjoy is key too. For example, I find going to the gym boring, but give me a zumba class and I will happily join in several times a week. It's all about finding what you like to keep you powering on.

I hope you've found my Intro useful, thank you so much again for buying my book, following me through the years and sharing your incredible support. I really hope you enjoy cooking my new recipes, that *Slimming Eats* inspires you to get in the kitchen, fall in love with real food and ingredients and start or keep going on your journey. Most of all, I want this way of eating to bring you a little bit more happiness and confidence in your daily life and ultimately, get you closer to achieving your goals, whatever they may be. If you have any questions at all, please do get in touch and tag me with your creations at #SlimmingEats – I can't wait to hear from you!

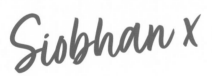

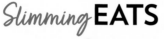

SlimmingEats.com   /SlimmingEatsRecipes   @SlimmingEats   @SlimmingEats

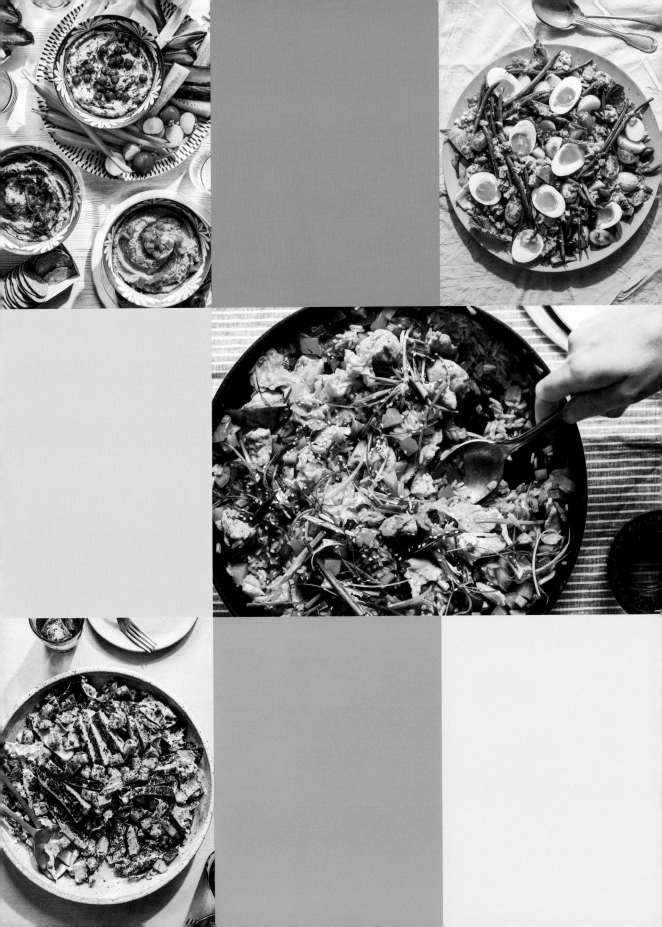

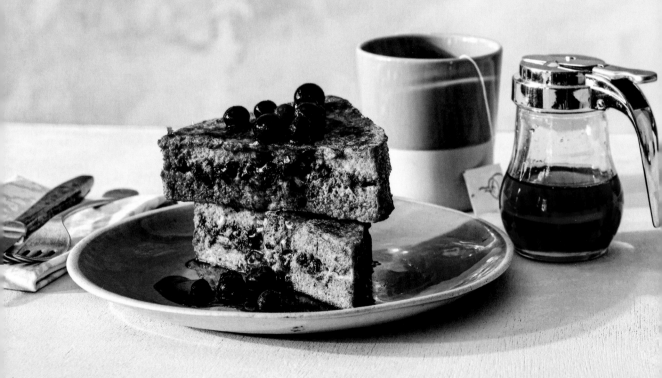

Breakfasts

Fruity Chia
Pudding with Vanilla
Greek Yoghurt

Mushroom and Spinach
Skillet with Eggs

Make-ahead Sausage,
Egg and Cheese
English Muffins

Breakfast Quiche
with Sweet Potato
Hash Brown Crust

Poached Egg
Breakfast Bowls with
Homemade Bagel
Seasoning

Breakfast Hash
Brown Roll

Baked Oats

Cheesy Scrambled
Eggs with Avocado
and Tomatoes

Overnight Pumpkin
Steel-cut Oats

Healthy Granola

Huevos Rancheros
with Chorizo-style
Minced Pork

Blueberry Cream
Cheese-stuffed
French Toast

190 Calories

Fruity Chia Pudding with Vanilla Greek Yoghurt

V

GF

KCALS
190

FAT
2.6g

SAT FAT
0.3g

CARBS
25.0g

SUGARS
23.2g

FIBRE
6.5g

PROTEIN
12.6g

SALT
0.12g

SERVES 3

150g (5½oz) frozen
   mixed berries
seeds of 1 pomegranate
120ml (4fl oz) pineapple
   juice
½ tablespoon lime juice
20g (¾oz) chia seeds
300g (10½oz) fat-free
   Greek yoghurt
1 teaspoon vanilla extract
2 tablespoons maple syrup
   (or honey)

Optional add-ins:
Top with a little sprinkle
of healthy granola
(see page 52).

Dairy-free:
Use dairy-free yoghurt
of choice.

A juicy and refreshing combination of mixed berries and pomegranate chia pudding spooned over slightly sweetened vanilla Greek yoghurt – perfect for breakfast or dessert.

1. In a bowl combine the frozen berries, pomegranate seeds, pineapple juice, lime juice and chia seeds. Cover and refrigerate overnight to allow to thicken.

2. Mix the yoghurt with the vanilla and maple syrup.

3. Serve the yoghurt in glasses and top with the fruit chia pudding.

4. Enjoy!

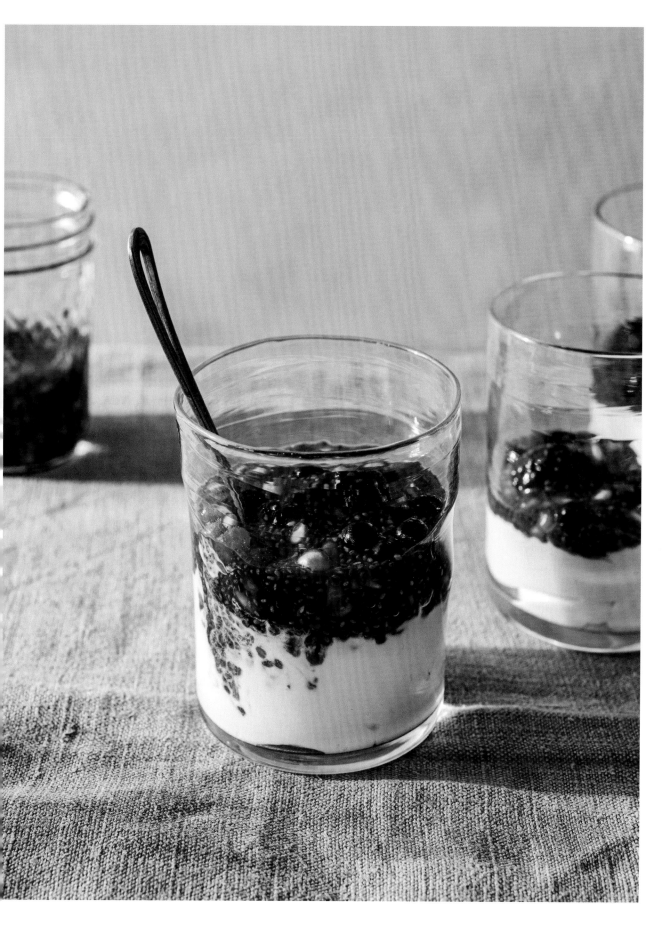

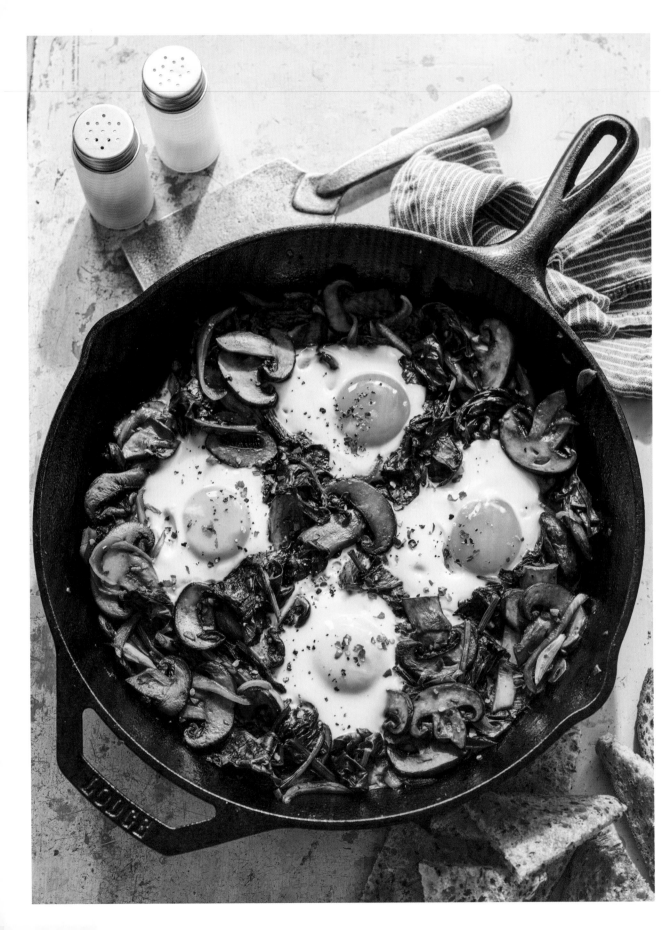

Mushroom and Spinach Skillet with Eggs

152 Calories

SERVES 4

1 tablespoon butter
300g (10½oz) mushrooms,
  sliced
1 small onion, halved and
  thinly sliced
salt and freshly ground
  black pepper
4 garlic cloves, minced
1 tablespoon balsamic
  vinegar
225g (8oz) spinach,
  washed and chopped
4 large eggs
pinch of red chilli flakes
  (optional)

Dairy-free:
Swap the butter for olive oil.

An easy all-in-one breakfast skillet of buttery garlic mushrooms, wilted spinach and delicious, perfectly cooked eggs. Simple enough just as it is or with some toast of your choice.

1. Melt the butter in a large skillet over a medium–high heat.

2. Add the mushrooms and onion and cook for about 10 minutes, until really golden. Season with a pinch of salt and freshly ground black pepper.

3. Add the garlic and cook for a further 30 seconds.

4. Add the balsamic vinegar and cook until it reduces down.

5. Add the spinach and cook until it wilts down, then make 4 wells in the mushroom and spinach mix and crack in the eggs.

6. Put a lid on the pan, reduce the heat to medium, and cook until the eggs are lightly set over the top but the yolks are still runny (unless you prefer a more cooked yolk).

7. Season the eggs with salt and freshly ground black pepper and add a pinch of chilli flakes, if you like.

8. Enjoy as it is, or serve with your favourite toast, some golden roasted potato cubes or sausage/bacon.

V

GF

KCALS
152

FAT
9.4g

SAT FAT
3.6g

CARBS
3.5g

SUGARS
2.6g

FIBRE
2.7g

PROTEIN
11.9g

SALT
0.52g

Make-ahead Sausage, Egg and Cheese English Muffins

KCALS
429

FAT
18.6g

SAT FAT
7.9g

CARBS
24.3g

SUGARS
6.9g

FIBRE
4.8g

PROTEIN
38.6g

SALT
2.19g

MAKES 8 BREAKFAST MUFFINS

olive oil spray
8 wholemeal (whole wheat) English muffins
8 large eggs
salt and freshly ground black pepper
8 slices of mature Cheddar (approx. 20g/¾oz each) – or American cheese slices

For the sausage patties:
800g (1lb 12oz) extra lean (5% fat) pork mince
2½ tablespoons water
1½ tablespoons chopped fresh sage
2 teaspoons paprika
1¼ teaspoons fine salt
½ teaspoon freshly ground black pepper
½ teaspoon fennel seeds, crushed in a pestle and mortar (optional)
pinch of red chilli flakes, (optional)
½ teaspoon onion powder
1 tablespoon maple syrup

Optional add-ins:
You can add some extra fillings, such as ketchup, spinach, tomato, avocado or leftover ajvar from page 136.

Swaps:
You can swap the sausage for ham or cooked bacon.

When it comes to mornings and work, we can often be pushed for time to make a decent filling breakfast. It's so easy to grab something quick and unhealthy instead, especially when we are tired and feeling uninspired. These make-ahead sausage, egg and cheese English muffins are ideal for those busy mornings – just grab, heat up and it's all ready to be enjoyed.

1. Combine the ingredients for the sausage patties together in a bowl and form into 8 equal-sized patties – you need to make them wider than the muffins, as they will shrink a little when cooked. I use a burger press to form perfectly round patties.

2. Place a frying pan over a medium–high heat and spray with olive oil, then cook the patties in 2 batches (I cook 4 at a time), until golden on both sides and cooked through (approx. 5–6 minutes per side).

3. Remove and set aside to cool.

4. Lightly toast the muffins and set aside to cool.

5. Pour approx. 0.5cm (¼ inch) of water into a frying pan (skillet) and place over a medium heat. Add 4 egg rings and, once the water is gently bubbling, crack the eggs into the rings. Add the lid and cook until the eggs are just set on top, but the yolks are still soft, then carefully remove, season with salt and freshly ground black pepper and allow to cool. Repeat with the 4 remaining eggs, using the same method (if most of the water has evaporated, add a little more to fill the bottom of the pan).

6. Once the ingredients have cooled you can build your muffins. Lay 8 muffin halves on a tray or large plate, add a slice of cheese to each muffin, top with a sausage patty, then the egg, and add the muffin tops. Wrap in parchment paper or foil, then these can either be kept in the fridge for up to 4 days or frozen.

7. Just take a muffin out as you want it and heat it in the oven or microwave. For the microwave, I wrap it in kitchen paper and heat at 30-second intervals until heated through (usually 1 minute from fridge or 3 minutes from freezer, but timings will vary according to microwave wattage), or you can wrap it in foil, place on a baking tray and heat in a 180°C/160°C fan/350°F/gas 4 oven for 15–20 minutes.

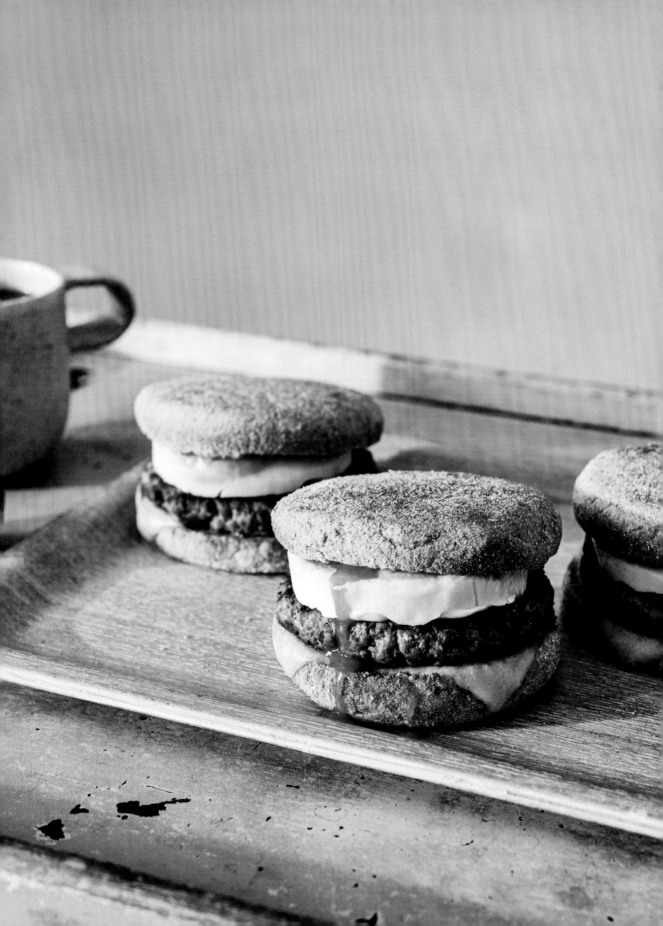

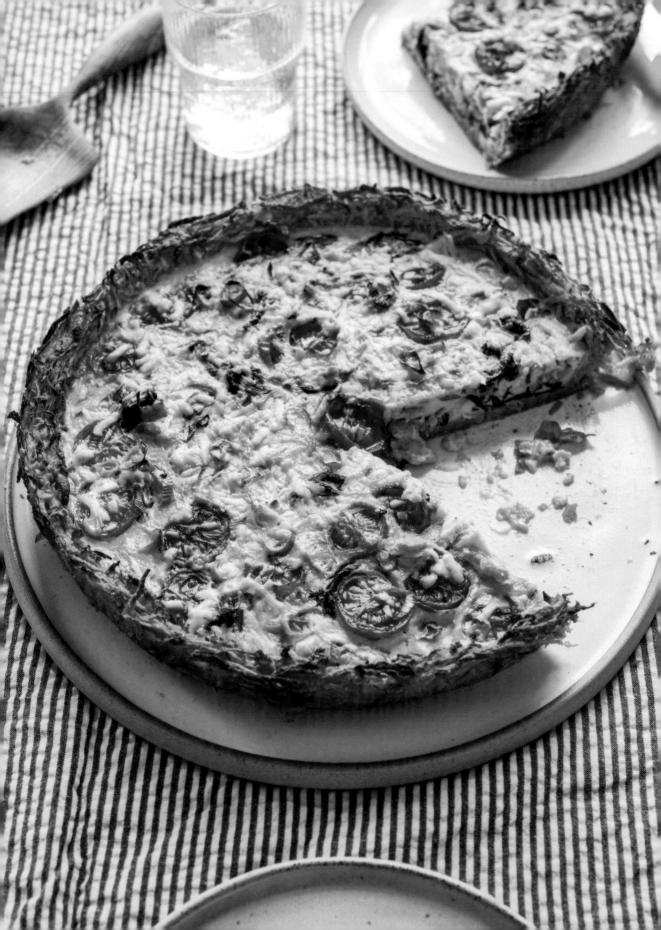

Breakfast Quiche with Sweet Potato Hash Brown Crust

GF

SERVES 6

For the base:
500g (1lb 2oz) sweet
   potatoes
2 teaspoons paprika
½ teaspoon garlic powder
½ teaspoon onion powder
50g (2oz) Parmesan, or
   vegetarian Italian-style hard
   cheese, grated
cooking oil spray

For the filling:
6 slices of lean back bacon
   (fat removed), chopped
100g (3½oz) spinach
15 cherry tomatoes, halved
200g (7oz) fat-free
   cottage cheese
6 large eggs
salt and freshly ground
   black pepper
30g (1oz) Cheddar,
   finely grated
1 spring onion (scallion),
   chopped

Variations:
You can really change this
up by adding different fillings
of your choice. Sausage is an
easy addition, or mushrooms,
peppers, etc., but I
recommend sautéing any
vegetables that could release
moisture before adding them
to the egg filling.
If you don't want to use
cheese, you can bind the
sweet potato hash brown
crust together with a couple
of egg whites.

This quiche is a great make-ahead filling breakfast. Delicious golden bacon, spinach and fresh tomato egg filling in a sweet potato hash brown crust.

1. Preheat the oven to 220°C/200°C fan/425°F/gas 7.

2. Peel and grate the sweet potatoes, then put them into a bowl with the paprika, garlic powder, onion powder and Parmesan and mix together to combine.

3. Grease a round 25cm (10 inch) ovenproof dish or quiche pan with cooking oil spray.

4. Add the sweet potato mix and pack it into the bottom and up round the sides. Don't worry if the mix feels dry and as if it won't hold together (as it bakes the cheese will melt, which binds it all).

5. Bake for about 18–20 minutes, until lightly golden.

6. While the base is baking, put the bacon into a pan and fry until golden, then remove and set aside. Add the spinach to the pan and cook until it just wilts, then remove and set aside.

7. Add the cherry tomatoes, cut side down, and sear in the pan just until lightly golden, then set those aside.

8. Put the cottage cheese and eggs into a blender and blend just until smooth.

9. Once the base is ready, pour in the egg/cottage cheese mix. Add the spinach and stir around to distribute evenly. Scatter in the tomatoes and bacon and season with a little salt and freshly ground black pepper.

10. Sprinkle over the grated Cheddar and chopped spring onion, then place in the oven and bake for 20 minutes at 200°C/180°C fan/400°F/gas 6.

11. The egg mixture should be golden and set. Let the quiche cool for 10 minutes before slicing to serve.

KCALS	**317**
FAT	**15.5g**
SAT FAT	**6.3g**
CARBS	**19.4g**
SUGARS	**6.9g**
FIBRE	**3.9g**
PROTEIN	**23.1g**
SALT	**1.66g**

Poached Egg Breakfast Bowls with Homemade Bagel Seasoning

V

DF

GF

KCALS
316

FAT
12.1g

SAT FAT
2.7g

CARBS
32.3g

SUGARS
6.2g

FIBRE
6.9g

PROTEIN
16.0g

SALT
1.20g

SERVES 2

For the bagel seasoning:
3 tablespoons toasted
  sesame seeds
2 tablespoons black
  sesame seeds
2 tablespoons dried
  onion flakes
2 tablespoons dried
  garlic flakes
2 tablespoons sea salt flakes
1½ tablespoons poppy seeds

*For the poached egg
breakfast bowl:*
1 x 400g (14oz) potato
½ small red onion, diced
½ tablespoon olive oil
½ teaspoon paprika
½ teaspoon onion powder
¼ teaspoon garlic powder
salt and freshly ground
  black pepper
175g (6oz) asparagus,
  trimmed
150g (5½oz) cherry
  tomatoes, halved
olive oil spray
2 large fresh eggs
2 handfuls of rocket (arugula)
  – approx. 25g (1oz)

Optional:
For a special occasion, add
cooked bacon, avocado or
smoked salmon. You can also
swap the rocket for micro
greens or cress. Yum!

Gluten-free:
Make sure the seeds/
seasonings/dried onion flakes
are free from gluten.

**These mouthwatering, colourful and healthy breakfast bowls
are fab for the weekend. Poached eggs with seasoned home fries,
roasted asparagus and tomatoes on a bed of rocket, finished off
with my bagel seasoning inspired by Trader Joe's Everything but
the Bagel Seasoning. I love this stuff, and it's so easy to make.
Store the rest of the seasoning blend in a jar and enjoy it on
everything from smoked salmon, avocado and tomatoes, to my
all-time breakfast favourite – eggs, cooked any way you like. It
will be a staple in your cupboard.**

1. To make the bagel seasoning, combine the ingredients in a bowl
and store in an airtight jar (you will only use a small pinch on the
breakfast bowl).

2. Pierce the potato and microwave for 5 minutes (If you don't have
a microwave, cut the potato into cubes and parboil until fork tender,
then drain and pat completely dry). Cut the potato into cubes and
put them into a bowl with the onion, the olive oil, paprika, onion
powder, garlic powder and a pinch of salt, and toss to coat.

3. Preheat the oven to 220°C/200°C fan/425°F/gas 7. Line a large
baking tray with parchment paper.

4. Spread the potatoes out on one side of the baking tray and bake
for 25–30 minutes, until golden. When there are 15 minutes
remaining, add the asparagus and tomatoes to the other half of the
tray, spray over the top with the olive oil spray and season with a
pinch of salt and freshly ground black pepper.

5. When the vegetables are almost cooked, you can poach the eggs.
Bring a small saucepan of water to the boil, then turn down the heat
so it is gently bubbling. Crack one egg at a time into a shallow bowl,
lower the edge of the bowl into the water, then carefully tip them
into the water (perfect cheat's method for poached eggs). Cook
for approx. 3 minutes, then lift with a slotted spatula and carefully
transfer to kitchen paper to absorb any excess water.

6. To build your poached egg breakfast bowl, put some rocket
(arugula) into each bowl, then some potatoes, tomatoes and
roasted asparagus (I slice it in half). Add a poached egg and finish
off the bowl by adding a pinch (or two) of the bagel seasoning.

7. Dig in and enjoy.

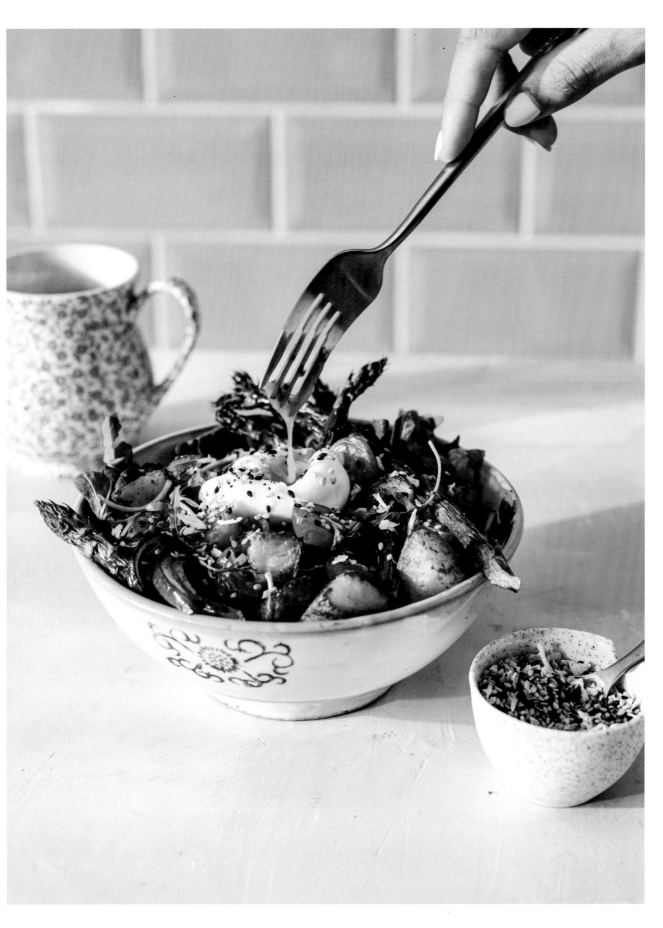

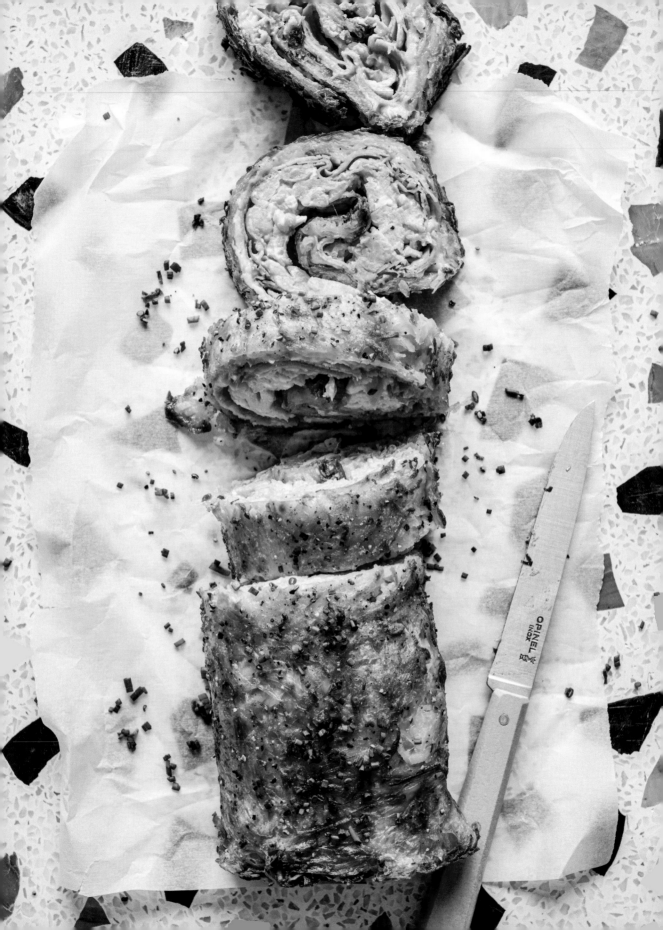

Breakfast Hash Brown Roll

SERVES 4

850g (1lb 14oz) floury
   potatoes (I use russets),
   peeled
salt and freshly ground
   black pepper
½ teaspoon onion powder
cooking oil spray
5 large eggs, beaten
100g (3½oz) mature
   Cheddar, freshly grated
6 slices of lean ham
chopped fresh chives,
   to sprinkle

Vegetarian:
Swap the ham for vegetables
of your choice, such as
spinach or the balsamic
tomatoes below.

Balsamic tomatoes:
These make a delicious side
to the hash brown roll. Just
sauté 1 small onion in cooking
oil spray until golden, add
some halved cherry or grape
tomatoes, then, just as the
tomatoes soften, add a
splash of balsamic vinegar
and season with salt and
freshly ground black pepper.

Kid-friendly option:
My kids love a slice of this
served with baked beans.

Variation:
Try a different cheese, like
Red Leicester.

A cheesy, golden hash brown roll-up filled with lean ham, Cheddar and scrambled eggs. A recipe for the whole family to enjoy! You can even play around with the filling by swapping out the ham for bacon, or adding in some sautéed veggies, like mushrooms or peppers.

1. Put the whole potatoes into a saucepan, cover with water and add a pinch of salt.

2. Bring to the boil, then turn off the heat but leave the potatoes in the water for 5 minutes.

3. Drain the potatoes fully and allow to cool slightly, then grate on to a clean tea towel and blot dry.

4. Put the grated potatoes into a bowl with 1 teaspoon of salt, onion powder and a pinch of freshly ground black pepper.

5. Preheat the oven to 220°C/200°C fan/425°F/gas 7.

6. Line a 30 x 23cm (12 x 9 inch) baking tray with parchment paper and spray with the cooking oil spray. Add the potato mixture and flatten it down across the whole tray, ensuring you compact it together as you do. Spray the oil over the top.

7. Place in the oven and bake for 30 minutes, then remove from oven, place a board over the tray and carefully flip. Place the paper back on the tray, then carefully slide the hash brown back on to the tray and bake for another 30 minutes, until golden all over.

8. When the hash brown is almost ready, put the beaten eggs into a non-stick saucepan and place over a low heat, stirring at intervals until the eggs are creamy and silky in appearance (but slightly undercooked).

9. Take the hash brown out of the oven. Add the cheese, then layer with the ham and lastly the scrambled eggs. Season with salt and freshly ground black pepper.

10. Starting at the short end of the sheet of hash brown, carefully roll it up into a large roll.

11. Put back into the oven for about 5 minutes, until the cheese is melted.

12. Sprinkle with chopped chives, cut into slices and enjoy!

GF

KCALS
396

FAT
17.1g

SAT FAT
7.8g

CARBS
32.9g

SUGARS
1.9g

FIBRE
3.9g

PROTEIN
25.6g

SALT
3.0g

Baked Oats

KCALS
328

FAT
10.1g

SAT FAT
2.3g

CARBS
37.4g

SUGARS
9.4g

FIBRE
3.1g

PROTEIN
18.0g

SALT
0.87g

SERVES 1

For the basic oats:
cooking oil spray
40g (1½ oz) oats
½ teaspoon baking powder
1 tablespoon granulated
    sweetener (or honey/maple
    syrup)
1 teaspoon flavouring
    (vanilla extract
    or ½ teaspoon ground
    spice such as cinnamon)
100g (3½oz) plain fat-free
    yoghurt
1 large egg

Gluten-free:
Use gluten-free oats and
baking powder

Dairy-free:
Use a dairy-free yoghurt.

Optional topping:
Enjoy with some fat-free
yoghurt of choice.

Who doesn't love cake for breakfast? Because, let's be honest, baked oats is pretty much a healthier version of cake, right? You can even make this the night before to save time and just warm it up in the morning. Below are some flavour ideas. The basic baked oats recipe is the same, just change your add-ins or flavours to make many different variations.

1. Preheat the oven to 190°C/170°C fan/375°F/gas 5.

2. Grease a round ovenproof dish about 12cm (5 inches) in diameter with oil spray.

3. Combine the dry ingredients in a bowl.

4. Combine the wet ingredients and fold them into the dry ingredients until combined.

5. Place in the greased dish, add your toppings if using, and bake for 30 minutes or until a skewer inserted in the centre comes out clean.

Ginger peach baked oats: Put 80g (3oz) of tinned peaches in syrup into a greased baking dish, then add your baked oats mix. Sprinkle the top with a crushed ginger snap biscuit and bake as above.

KCALS	FAT	SAT FAT	CARBS	SUGARS	FIBRE	PROTEIN	SALT
421	11.6g	3.0g	55.4g	23.0g	4.3g	18.9g	1.13g

Strawberry banana and chocolate baked oats: Put the basic baked oats mix into a greased baking dish. Scatter over 40g (1½oz) of chopped banana, 3 chopped strawberries and 5g (⅛oz) of chocolate chips and bake as above.

KCALS	FAT	SAT FAT	CARBS	SUGARS	FIBRE	PROTEIN	SALT
406	12.2g	3.4g	49.7g	20.2g	5.5g	19.0g	1.02g

Carrot cake oats: Add ½ teaspoon of ground cinnamon and ¼ teaspoon of ground ginger to the basic baked oats mix, then fold in some orange zest, 35g (1¼oz) of finely grated carrot and 10g (¼oz) of sultanas. Put into a greased baking dish, sprinkle over 5g (⅛oz) of chopped walnuts, and bake as above.

KCALS	FAT	SAT FAT	CARBS	SUGARS	FIBRE	PROTEIN	SALT
416	13.8g	2.7g	48.0g	18.8g	6.1g	19.5g	1.05g

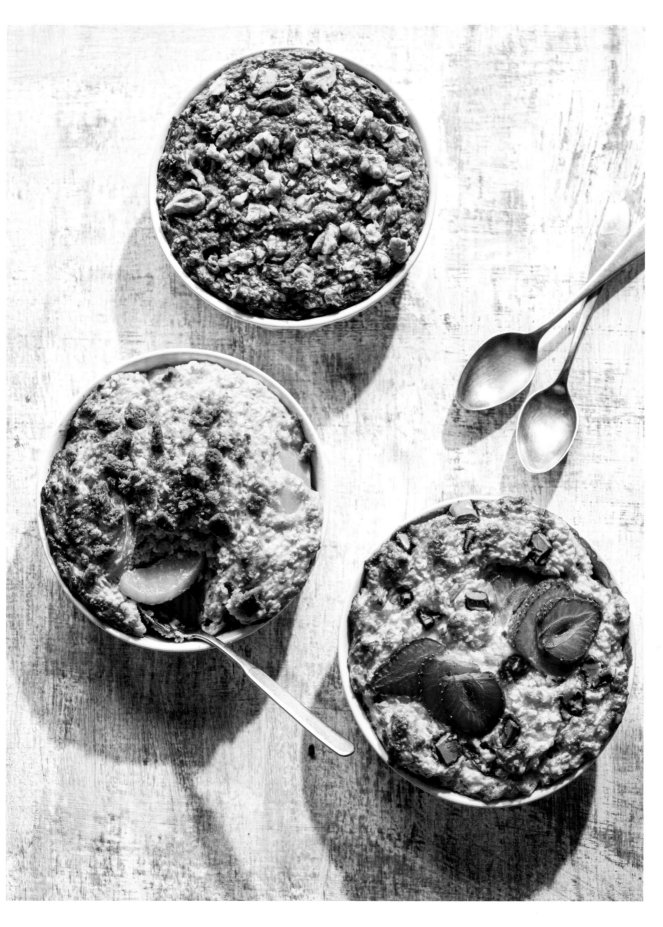

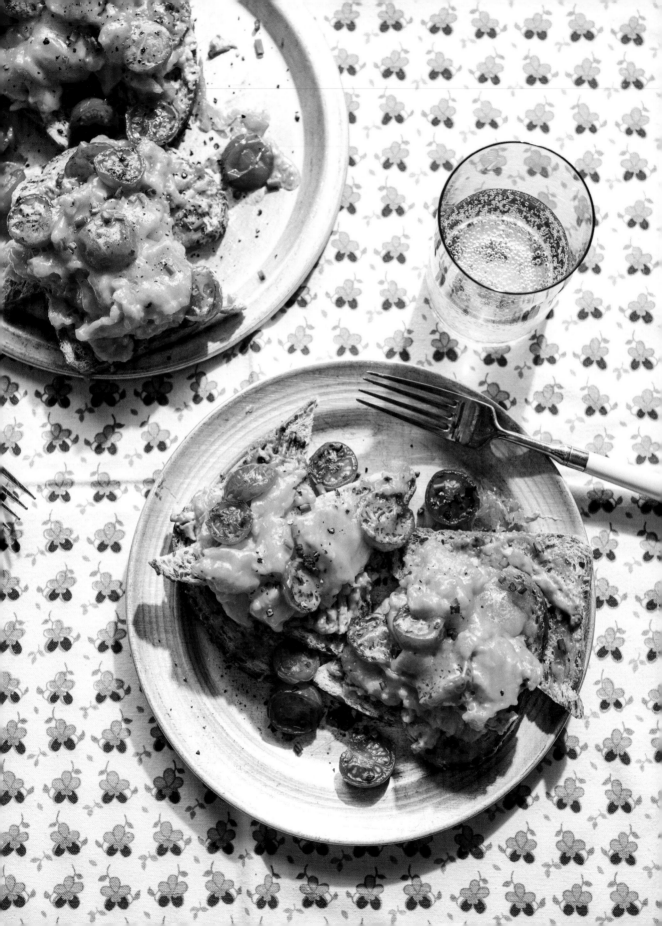

Cheesy Scrambled Eggs with Avocado and Tomatoes

438 Calories

SERVES 2

cooking oil spray
12 cherry tomatoes, halved
90g (3oz) avocado
sea salt and freshly ground
   black pepper
4 slices of low-calorie
   wholemeal (whole wheat)
   bread
4 large eggs
30g (1oz) Red Leicester,
   grated
chopped fresh chives or
   spring onions (scallions),
   green part only

Gluten-free:
Use gluten-free bread.

My favourite breakfast combo! Creamy scrambled eggs and mashed avocado on toast, scattered with slightly softened cherry tomatoes and Red Leicester cheese, then finished off under the grill.

1. Spray a frying pan with the cooking oil, then add the tomatoes, cut side down, and lightly brown them. Carefully flip them over and brown the skin side (so the tomatoes are slightly softened). Set aside.

2. Put the avocado into a bowl and mash with a pinch of salt.

3. Toast the bread lightly until golden. Cut each slice into 2 triangles and spread the avocado over each one. Place the toast on a baking tray in 2 sections (so 4 triangles) for each serving, slightly overlapping each toast triangle.

4. Crack the eggs into a small saucepan and whisk until combined. Place on a low–medium heat and stir intermittently, removing from the heat as you do so, until the eggs are creamy and silky in appearance.

5. Top the avocado toast with the eggs, scatter over the softened tomatoes, add the grated cheese, and place under the grill until the cheese is just melted.

6. Carefully transfer each section on to a plate using a spatula. Sprinkle with chopped chives or spring onions (scallions) and season with salt and freshly ground black pepper.

V

KCALS
438

FAT
27.0g

SAT FAT
8.5g

CARBS
19.6g

SUGARS
3.6g

FIBRE
6.0g

PROTEIN
26.1g

SALT
1.16g

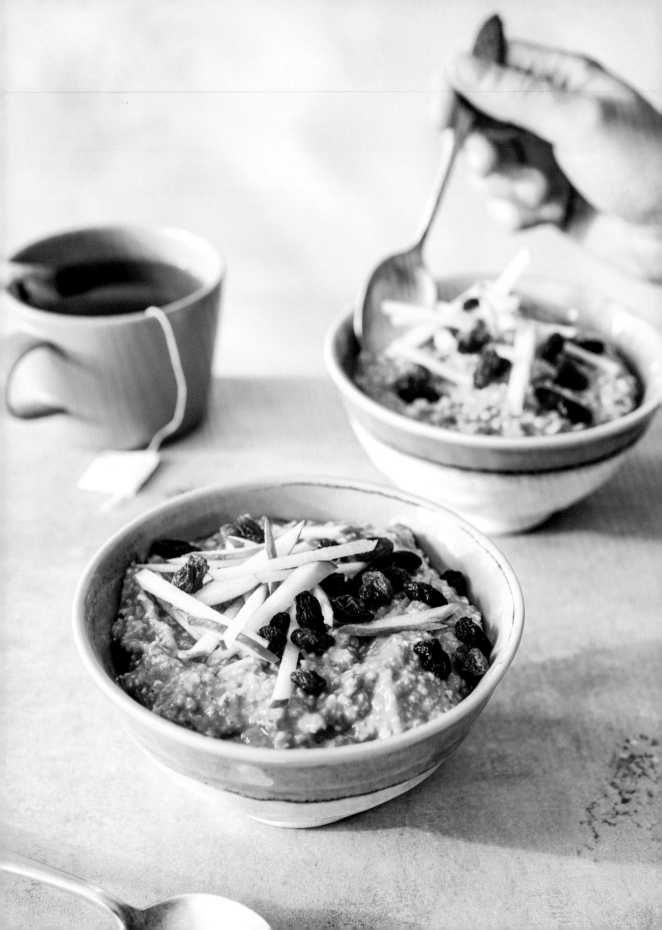

Overnight Pumpkin Steel-cut Oats

V

SERVES 4

1 tablespoon butter
250g (9oz) tinned
  pumpkin purée
4 tablespoons Demerara
  sugar
½ teaspoon ground
  cinnamon
¼ teaspoon ground ginger
¼ teaspoon grated nutmeg
160g (6oz) steel-cut oats
  (also called pinhead or
  Irish oats)
600ml (20fl oz) water
a little splash of milk of
  your choice
pinch of salt

My favourite toppings:
2 crisp sweet apples, diced
40g (1½oz) sultanas

This overnight oats recipe is a simple prep-the-night-before-and-forget-about-it-until-the-morning recipe that the whole family will love. Buttery cinnamon brown sugar pumpkin purée with delicious nutty steel-cut oats – the only difficult part is deciding which toppings to add.

1. Melt the butter in a small saucepan. Add the pumpkin purée, sugar and spices and cook until the pumpkin deepens in colour.

2. Stir in the oats and water, bring to the boil, then cover, turn off the heat and leave overnight.

3. In the morning, add a little milk of your choice to loosen the oats, heating and stirring until piping hot. Leftovers can be stored in a resealable tub in the fridge for the next morning.

4. Serve in bowls and top with diced apple and sultanas.

Dairy-free:
Use dairy-free milk
and butter.

Gluten-free:
Use gluten-free steel-cut/
pinhead oats.

Sugar swap:
If you prefer, you can swap
the Demerara sugar for a
brown granulated sweetener
of choice.

More topping suggestions:
Pumpkin seeds, blueberries,
diced pear, peach, banana,
nuts or nut butter. A little
sprinkling of healthy granola
(see page 52) is tasty too.

Substitute for tinned pumpkin:
Swap for an equal amount
of mashed sweet potato or
butternut squash.

KCALS
350

FAT
7.1g

SAT FAT
2.8g

CARBS
62.0g

SUGARS
33.1g

FIBRE
5.6g

PROTEIN
6.8g

SALT
0.10g

Healthy Granola

V

DF

KCALS
218

FAT
9.9g

SAT FAT
3.1g

CARBS
24.6g

SUGARS
8.9g

FIBRE
2.8g

PROTEIN
6.1g

SALT
0.12g

10 SERVINGS

200g (7oz) large oats
4 tablespoons raw
    pumpkin seeds
45 raw cashews, halved
30g (1½oz) sultanas
1 tablespoon ground
    cinnamon
pinch of salt
20g (¾oz) coconut oil
5 tablespoons maple syrup
    or honey
1 teaspoon vanilla extract
60ml (2fl oz) pineapple juice
1 large egg white

Gluten-free:
Use gluten-free oats.

Variations:
Try different nuts, seeds and
dried fruits for alternative
flavours.

As a family that loves granola, we tend to avoid store-bought brands, which can be packed with sugar and often contain a lot of calories for a measly serving. This homemade granola recipe uses simple healthy ingredients like oats, nuts and seeds, and is naturally sweetened with maple syrup and pineapple juice.

1. Preheat the oven to 180°C/160°C fan/350°F/gas 4. Place the oats, pumpkin seeds, cashews, sultanas, cinnamon and pinch of salt in a bowl.

2. Melt the coconut oil in the microwave (15 seconds), and whisk in the maple syrup, vanilla and pineapple juice. Whisk in the egg white.

3. Pour into the oat mixture and stir until combined.

4. Spread out the mixture in a thin layer on a baking tray lined with parchment paper.

5. Place in the oven and bake for 30–35 minutes, until golden.

6. Store in an airtight container for up to 2 weeks.

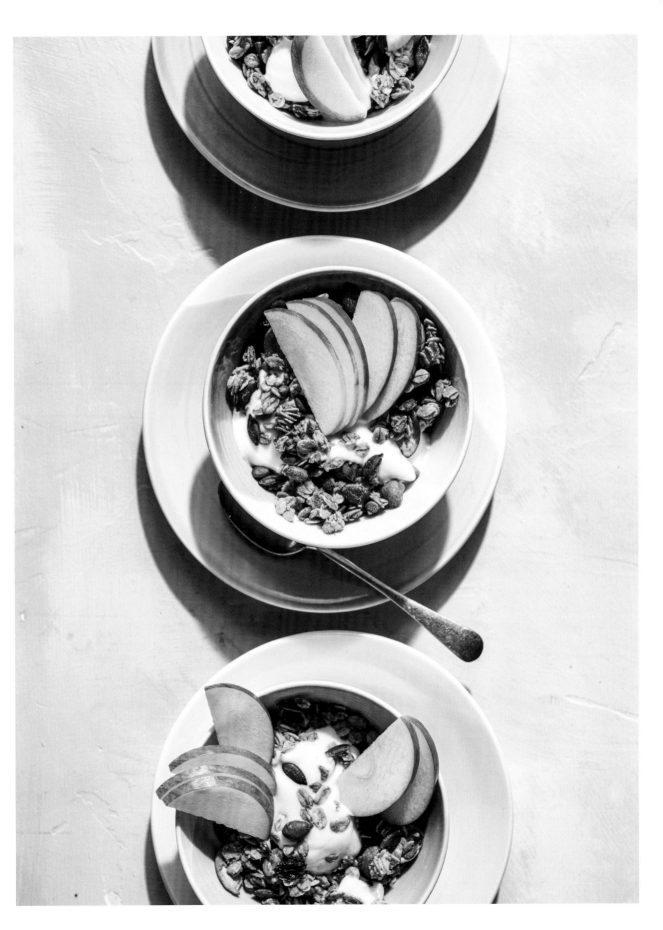

Huevos Rancheros with Chorizo-style Minced Pork

KCALS	**475**
FAT	**26.3g**
SAT FAT	**9.3g**
CARBS	**23.6g**
SUGARS	**7.5g**
FIBRE	**6.6g**
PROTEIN	**32.8g**
SALT	**1.7g**

SERVES 4

For the minced pork:
300g (10½oz) extra-lean
   (5% fat) pork mince
½ tablespoon maple syrup
1 tablespoon apple
   cider vinegar
¼ teaspoon cayenne pepper
1 tablespoon paprika
½ teaspoon smoked paprika
1 teaspoon ground cumin
1 teaspoon garlic powder
½ teaspoon dried thyme
½ teaspoon dried oregano
pinch of ground cinnamon
salt and freshly ground
   black pepper

For the rancheros sauce:
cooking oil spray
½ a small onion, finely diced
1 small jalapeño, deseeded
   and diced
1 garlic clove, crushed
1 x 400g (14oz) tin of
   chopped tomatoes
½ teaspoon ground cumin
¼ teaspoon dried oregano
¼ teaspoon salt
1 teaspoon chipotle
   chilli powder
couple of fresh coriander
   (cilantro) leaves
1 teaspoon lime juice
90ml (3fl oz) water

For the huevos rancheros:
4 low-calorie wholemeal
   (whole wheat) tortillas
4 eggs
60g (2oz) feta, crumbled
fresh coriander (cilantro)
1 small avocado, sliced

This yummy recipe is inspired by my favourite local breakfast café. Their version of the huevos rancheros combines homemade chorizo sausage with the standard rancheros sauce, avocado, feta, and a sunny-side-up egg over a warmed tortilla. It's heavenly!

1. To make the chorizo-style minced pork, mix the pork with the maple syrup (this helps with the caramelization of the pork), vinegar, spices and herbs. Place a frying pan over a medium–high heat and spray it with the cooking oil, then fry the pork until caramelized.

2. To make the rancheros sauce, heat some cooking oil spray in a small saucepan. Add the onion and jalapeño, and fry until softened.

3. Add the garlic and fry for a further 30 seconds. Add the tomatoes, seasonings and water, bring to the boil, then simmer covered for 8–10 minutes. Blend until smooth (or enjoy chunky).

4. Warm the tortillas in a pan with a little oil spray until they just start to blister on the surface. Set aside.

5. Spray the frying pan with cooking oil spray, crack in the eggs and cook to your preference (sunny side up – soft yolk – is my favourite).

6. Top each tortilla with pork mix, rancheros sauce, egg, crumbled feta, fresh coriander (cilantro) and avocado slices.

Vegetarian option:
Swap out the homemade
chorizo-style minced pork
for some black beans.

Gluten-free:
Use gluten-free wraps and
chipotle powder.

Lower-carb option:
Swap the wrap for double
sunny-side-up eggs.

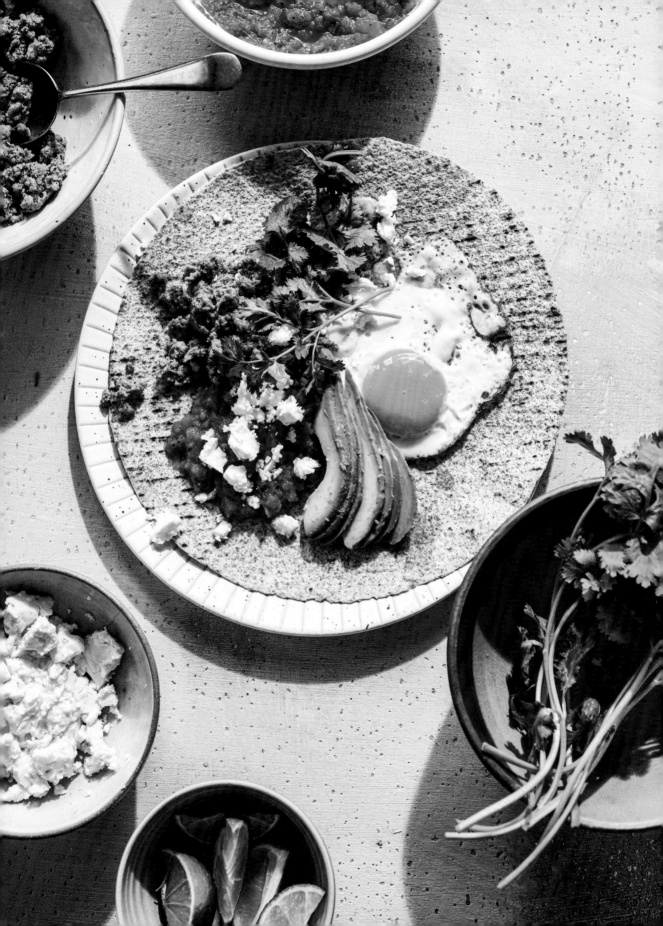

Blueberry Cream Cheese-stuffed French Toast

SERVES 2

200g (7oz) frozen
   blueberries
2 tablespoons maple syrup
2 tablespoons water
1 teaspoon lemon juice
4 tablespoons milk
2 eggs
1 teaspoon vanilla extract
1 tablespoon brown
   granulated sweetener
4 slices of low-calorie
   wholemeal (whole wheat)
   bread
45g (1½oz) light
   cream cheese
cooking oil spray

Gluten-free:
Use gluten-free bread
of choice.

Variation:
Try with different fruits such
as blackberries, strawberries,
cherries or raspberries.

Love French toast? This stuffed version takes it to a whole other level – scrumptious eggy bread stuffed with sweet blueberry coulis and cream cheese.

1. Put the blueberries into a small saucepan with 1 tablespoon of the maple syrup, the water and lemon juice and cook until they become soft and syrupy, roughly mashing them up in the pan (you want them to be almost jam-like, not too thick but not too liquidy either).

2. Whisk together the milk, eggs, vanilla and sweetener.

3. Slice each slice of bread in half on the diagonal so you have 8 triangles.

4 Spread 4 triangles with cream cheese and top with the cooked blueberries (only use about two-thirds of the blueberries, saving the rest for topping).

5. Place the other triangles on top, so you now have 4 blueberry cream cheese triangle sandwiches.

6. Place the sandwiches in the egg mixture, carefully turning them over to coat and ensure all the mixture is absorbed into the bread.

7. Heat a large frying pan on a medium heat and spray with the cooking oil.

8. Add the stuffed French toast and cook on one side until golden brown. Spray the top (uncooked side) with spray oil, then flip them over and repeat on the other side.

9. Serve on plates, topping with the remaining cooked blueberries and drizzling each plate with the rest of the maple syrup.

10. Enjoy!

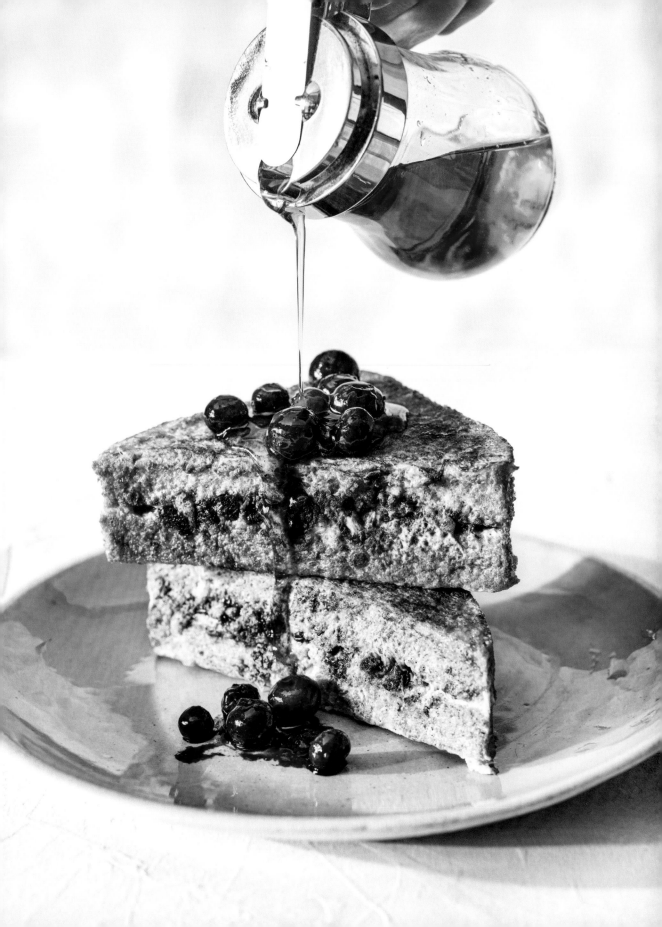

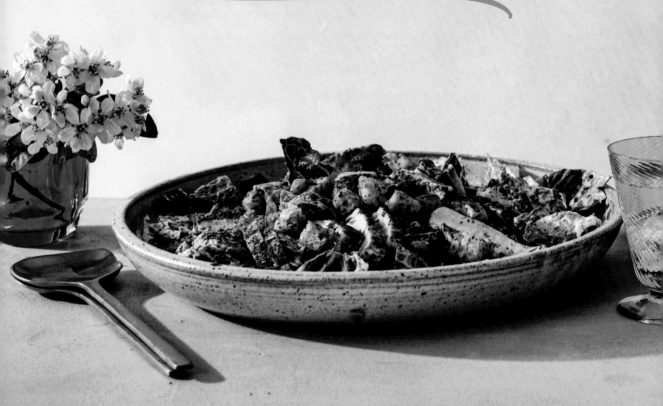

Soups and Salads

Turmeric, Chicken and
Cauliflower Soup

Garlicky White Bean,
Orzo and Spinach Soup

Curried Sweet Potato
and Lentil Soup

Pasta e Fagioli Soup

French Onion Soup

Chicken Corn Chowder

Ham, Vegetable and
Pearl Barley Soup

Spicy Turkey Meatballs
and Rice Soup

Chicken Dill Pickle Salad

BLT Pasta Salad

Tuna Niçoise Salad

Bacon, Peach and
Fennel Salad

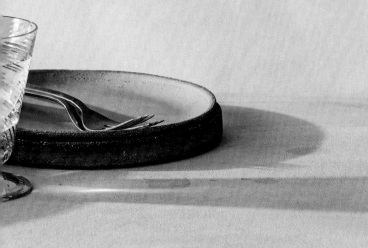

Turmeric, Chicken and Cauliflower Soup

GF

DF

KCALS
219

FAT
4.9g

SAT FAT
1.3g

CARBS
15.1g

SUGARS
10.2g

FIBRE
7.2g

PROTEIN
24.9g

SALT
1.53g

SERVES 4

cooking oil spray
1 onion, diced
100g (3½oz) celery, chopped
200g (7oz) carrots, halved lengthways and chopped into 2cm (¾ inch) chunks
250g (9oz) butternut squash, peeled and cubed
2 teaspoons grated fresh ginger
4 garlic cloves, crushed
1 teaspoon ground turmeric
900ml (1½ pints) chicken stock
300g (10½oz) cauliflower
300g (10½oz) skinless chicken breast, kept in large pieces
2 tablespoons chopped fresh coriander (cilantro)
salt

Optional:
Stir in a little coconut milk for added creaminess or add in some cooked rice for a more filling meal.

Vegetarian:
To make this vegetarian, swap the chicken stock for vegetable stock and use vegetables, beans or lentils instead of chicken.

Freezing:
To reheat after freezing, simply defrost in the fridge, then warm through in the microwave or in a saucepan over a medium heat.

A warming golden soup, delicately flavoured with turmeric, garlic and ginger and packed with vegetables, along with tender chicken, poached in stock for maximum flavour.

1. Place a deep saucepan on a medium heat and spray with cooking oil.

2. Add the onion, celery and carrots and fry for a few minutes to soften.

3. Add the squash, ginger and garlic and fry for another minute.

4. Add the turmeric and stir until coated.

5. Pour in the stock, then add the cauliflower and the chicken.

6. Bring to the boil, then cover and simmer for 20–25 minutes.

7. Remove the chicken from the pan and shred with a knife. Set aside.

8. Remove about 4 ladles of the veg along with a little of the broth and blend until smooth. Return this blended soup to the pan with the chicken and coriander (cilantro) and stir until it's all velvety and thickened.

9. Taste and season with a pinch of salt as needed.

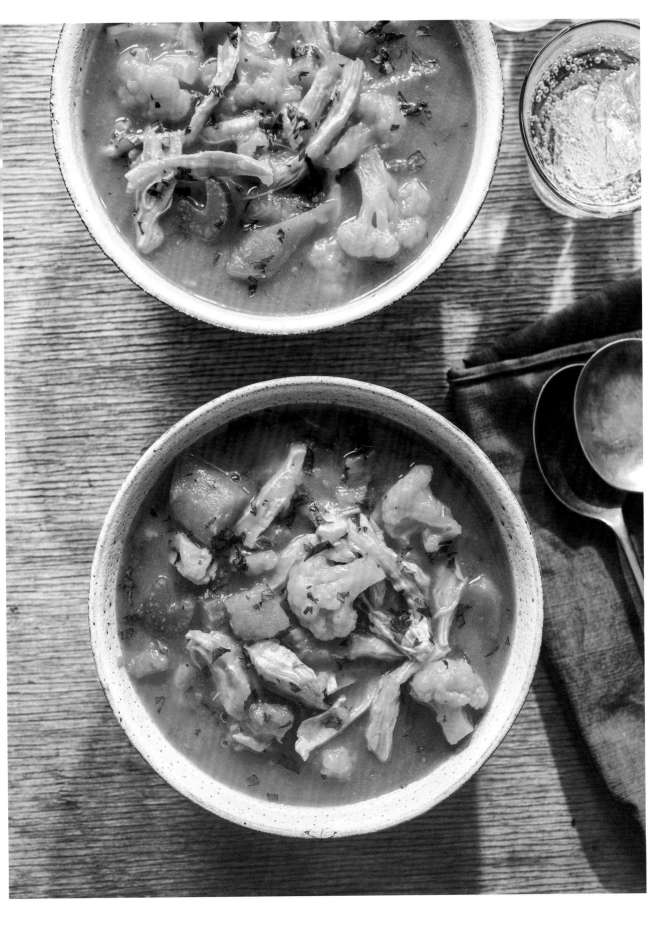

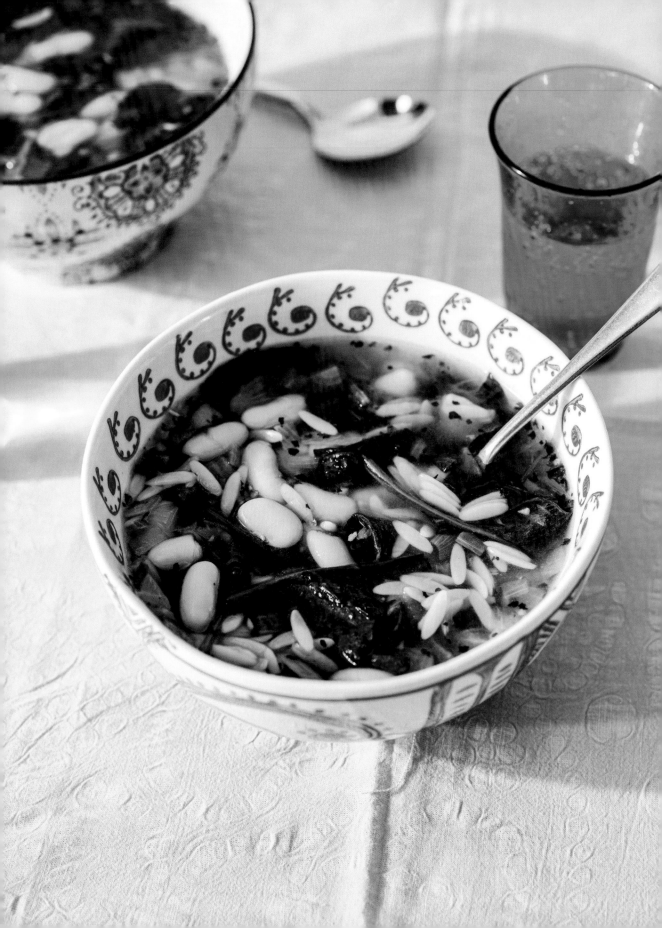

Garlicky White Bean, Orzo and Spinach Soup

SERVES 4

olive oil spray
2 onions, finely diced
salt and freshly ground
   black pepper
6 garlic cloves, crushed
675ml (22fl oz) vegetable
   stock
1 x 400g (14oz) tin of
   cannellini beans (white),
   drained and rinsed
½ teaspoon dried rosemary
½ teaspoon dried thyme
pinch of red chilli flakes
   (optional)
100g (3½oz) dried orzo pasta
2 big handfuls of spinach,
   stalks removed, roughly
   chopped

Gluten-free:
You could swap orzo for rice.

Additional toppings:
This soup is delicious
topped with cooked chicken
or bacon, or a little grated
cheese such as Parmesan or
mature Cheddar.

For a creamier texture:
Before adding the orzo,
roughly blend with a hand
blender (you want some
white beans left whole).

Freezing:
You could freeze the soup
after step 3. To reheat after
freezing, simply defrost in the
fridge, warm through over
a medium heat, then follow
steps 4–6.

A simple but delicious soup that comes loaded with flavour from six full cloves of garlic, herbs, orzo pasta and healthy spinach, with a silky, creamy finish from hearty, protein-rich white beans.

1. Place a frying pan over a medium–high heat and spray with the olive oil. Add the onions and a pinch of salt and fry for a couple of minutes.

2. Add the garlic, then gradually add 180ml (6fl oz) of the stock, reducing it down with each addition, until the garlic and onions are softened, lightly caramelized and sweetened.

3. Add the cannellini beans, herbs, chilli flakes (if using) and the rest of the stock, bring to the boil, then simmer for 10 minutes.

4. In the meantime cook the orzo according to the package instructions (al dente).

5. Stir in the cooked orzo, then add the spinach and stir until wilted.

6. Taste and season with salt and freshly ground black pepper as needed.

212 Calories	
KCALS	**212**
FAT	**1.6g**
SAT FAT	**0.3g**
CARBS	**35.7g**
SUGARS	**6.3g**
FIBRE	**7.5g**
PROTEIN	**10.0g**
SALT	**0.53g**

Curried Sweet Potato and Lentil Soup

KCALS
328

FAT
9.9g

SAT FAT
6.8g

CARBS
45.3g

SUGARS
14.3g

FIBRE
12.8g

PROTEIN
8.1g

SALT
0.53g

SERVES 4

cooking oil spray
1 large onion, cut into
    small dice
½ tablespoon grated
    fresh ginger
3 garlic cloves, crushed
2 teaspoons ground cumin
2 teaspoons ground
    coriander
1 teaspoon ground turmeric
½ teaspoon hot chilli powder
600g (21oz) sweet potatoes,
    peeled and cubed
1 x 400g (14oz) tin of lentils,
    drained and rinsed
480ml (17fl oz) vegetable
    stock
1 x 400ml (14fl oz) tin of
    light coconut milk
salt
2–3 tablespoons chopped
    fresh coriander (cilantro)

Gluten-free:
Use gluten-free chilli powder.

Freezing:
To reheat after freezing,
simply defrost in the fridge
and warm through in the
microwave or in a saucepan
over a medium heat.

This curried sweet potato and lentil soup is probably one of my favourite meat-free soups that I make on regular rotation. We love sweet potato, and it adds a subtle sweetness against the spices and creaminess of the coconut milk.

1. Place a large saucepan over a medium–high heat and spray with cooking oil.

2. Add the onion and fry until golden and translucent.

3. Add the ginger and garlic, and fry until the garlic just starts to go golden (add a little water to prevent burning if needed). Add the spices and stir until it becomes paste-like.

4. Add the sweet potatoes, lentils, stock and light coconut milk. Bring to the boil, then simmer for 15 minutes, until the sweet potato is softened. Roughly crush some of the sweet potato to help thicken the soup.

5. Taste and season with salt as needed, then stir in the fresh coriander.

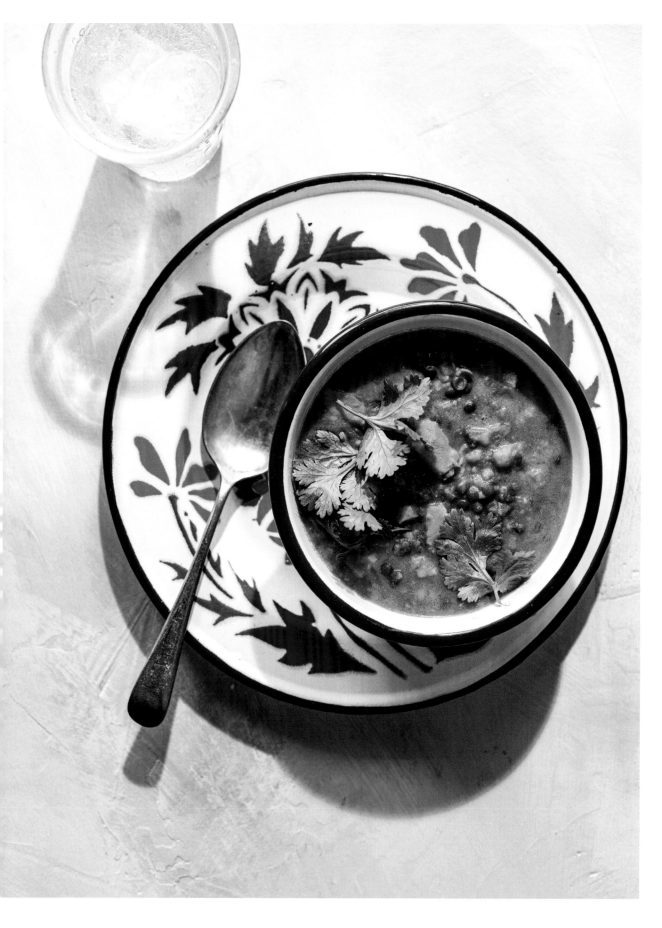

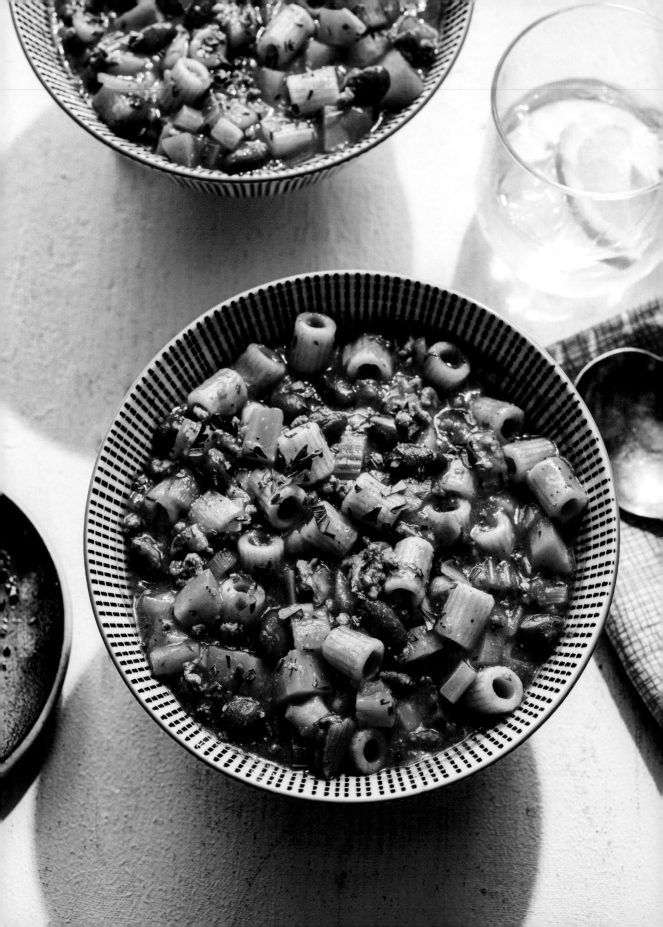

Pasta e Fagioli Soup

SERVES 6

olive oil spray
400g (14oz) extra lean
(5% fat) beef mince
150g (5½oz) onion, diced
150g (5½oz) celery, diced
150g (5½oz) carrots, diced
4 garlic cloves, crushed
1½ tablespoons dried mixed
(Italian) herbs
1 x 400g (14oz) tin of
chopped tomatoes
5 tablespoons tomato purée
(paste)
720ml (1¼ pints) beef stock
720ml (1¼ pints) chicken
stock
1 x 400g (14oz) tin of kidney
beans, drained and rinsed
1 x 400g (14oz) tin of
cannellini (white) beans,
drained and rinsed
150g (5½oz) dried ditalini
pasta (tubetti), or other
soup-sized pasta
salt and freshly ground
black pepper
2–3 tablespoons chopped
fresh parsley

Optional:

Serve with a grating of
Parmesan (omit if dairy-free).

Swaps:

Turkey or chicken mince also
work well in this recipe or
you can use sausage meat if
you like.

Freezing:

You can freeze the soup after
step 4. To reheat, simply
defrost the soup in the fridge,
warm through over a medium
heat, then follow steps 5–7.

Occasionally I get together with my neighbour and we spend a day cooking a variety of different soups to stock up our freezers – and this one is often on our list. Pasta e fagioli is a popular recipe and it can be easily varied by using different minced meats (such as chicken or turkey), or even sausage. I like to use minced beef, along with two different beans for some additional protein, and little tubetti pasta (ditalini), but you really can add in any small soup pasta you like. It's a perfect filling meal in a bowl, and it's even nicer finished off with a little grating of Parmesan. Totally optional, of course.

1. Put a large saucepan on a medium heat and spray with olive oil.

2. Add the minced beef, onion, celery, carrots and garlic, and fry until the meat is browned and the vegetables are softened, breaking up any large pieces of meat.

3. Add the mixed herbs and stir to coat.

4. Add the tinned tomatoes, tomato purée, beef and chicken stock, bring to the boil, then reduce the heat and simmer for 20 minutes.

5. Add the drained beans and the pasta and continue to simmer until the pasta is cooked (approx. 7–8 minutes).

6. Taste and season as need with salt and freshly ground black pepper.

7. Stir in the chopped parsley and serve. If you are not eating straight away, the pasta will continue to absorb liquid, so you may want to add more stock before reheating if you prefer your soup more broth-like.

DF

KCALS
348

FAT
5.1g

SAT FAT
1.9g

CARBS
39.4g

SUGARS
9.1g

FIBRE
11.3g

PROTEIN
30.5g

SALT
1.07g

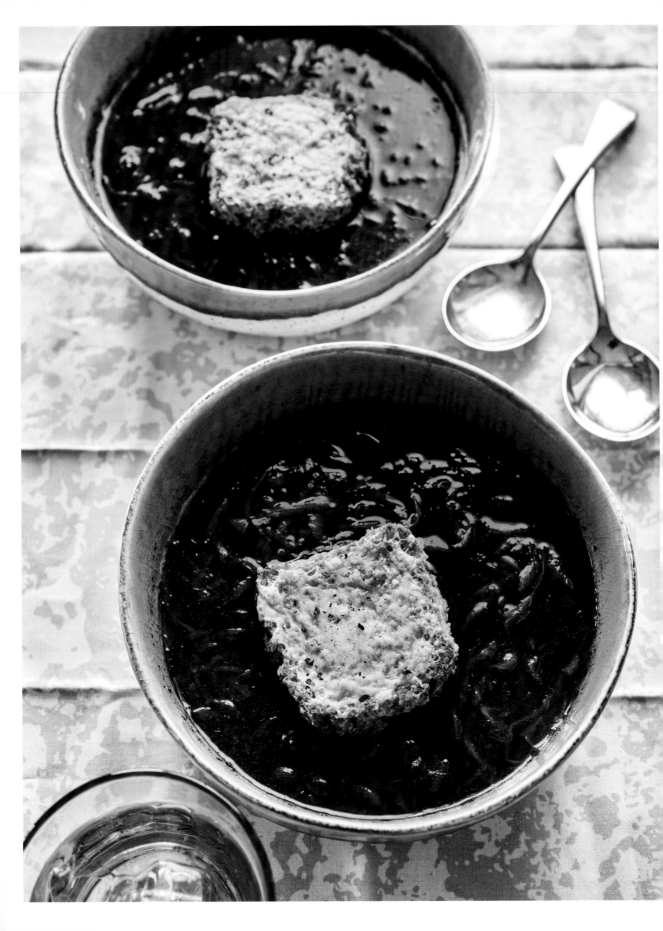

French Onion Soup

SERVES 4

½ tablespoon butter
½ tablespoon olive oil
900g (2lb) onions (I used
    450g/1lb white onions
    and 450g/1lb red onions),
    halved and thinly sliced
1 teaspoon maple syrup
salt and freshly ground
    black pepper
1.4 litres (2½ pints) beef
    stock
2 garlic cloves, crushed (plus
    an additional whole clove
    for rubbing over the bread)
1 teaspoon dried thyme
    (or a few sprigs of fresh)
1 tablespoon tomato purée
    (paste)
2 tablespoons balsamic
    vinegar
1 bay leaf
2 x 60g (2oz) wholemeal
    (whole wheat) rolls,
    split in half
cooking oil spray
60g (2oz) Gruyère (or other
    Swiss cheese), grated

Freezing:
Only the soup is suitable
for freezing. To reheat after
freezing, simply defrost the
soup in the fridge, then warm
through over a medium heat
or in the microwave. Prepare
the cheesy bread while you
reheat the soup.

Vegetarian:
Use vegetable stock, and
add that rich beefy flavour by
adding 2 teaspoons of yeast
extract (Marmite).

One of my favourite soups is French onion soup, but traditional recipes can pack in a whole heap of calories with all that crusty bread and cheese. This slightly healthier version still has all those amazing, rich flavours but far fewer calories.

1. Put the butter and olive oil into a deep saucepan and heat over a medium–high heat. Once hot, add the onions and sauté in the oil and butter for a couple of minutes until they start to go golden, then add the maple syrup and a pinch of freshly ground black pepper and stir to coat.

2. Add a little of the beef stock, put the lid on the pan, and let the onions cook for 20 minutes (don't try to skip or rush this process, as you won't get the rich flavours and caramelized colour of the onions). At intervals remove the lid, add a little more of the stock and stir to prevent burning. After 20 minutes the onions should be really caramelized and softened.

3. Add the crushed garlic, thyme, tomato purée and balsamic vinegar and continue to cook for just 1 minute.

4. Pour in the rest of the stock and add the bay leaf, then bring to the boil, cover the pan and simmer for 20 minutes.

5. Preheat the oven to 200°C/180°C fan/400°F/gas 6.

6. When the soup is almost ready, place the halved rolls on a baking tray lined with parchment paper. Spray the tops of the rolls with cooking oil, then cut the additional garlic clove in half and rub all over the bread. Bake for 10 minutes, until lightly golden and crispy.

7. Taste the soup and season as needed with salt and freshly ground black pepper, then ladle it into 4 oven-friendly bowls. Add one half bread roll to each bowl, top with a little Gruyère cheese, and bake for 10–12 minutes or place under the grill (broiler) until the cheese topping is all melted and golden.

KCALS
325

FAT
11.2g

SAT FAT
4.9g

CARBS
34.9g

SUGARS
17.8g

FIBRE
8.8g

PROTEIN
16.9g

SALT
0.96g

Chicken Corn Chowder

KCALS
322

FAT
10.7g

SAT FAT
4.4g

CARBS
24.9g

SUGARS
9.9g

FIBRE
4.5g

PROTEIN
29.2g

SALT
2.07g

SERVES 6

6 slices of lean bacon (fat removed), diced
1 tablespoon butter
160g (6oz) onions, diced
200g (7oz) carrots, diced
1 stalk of celery, diced
2 garlic cloves, crushed
1 red pepper, diced
400g (14oz) waxy potatoes, peeled and cubed
480ml (17fl oz) chicken stock
480ml (17fl oz) semi-skimmed milk
2 tablespoons cornflour (cornstarch)
300g (10½oz) cooked chicken, diced
160g (6oz) frozen sweetcorn
salt and freshly ground black pepper
chopped fresh chives

Freezing:
To reheat after freezing, simply defrost in the fridge and warm through in the microwave or in a saucepan over a medium heat.

This is a handy soup if you have some leftover cooked chicken to use. The chunks of vegetables in a light creamy broth are finished off with some golden bacon, it's pure comfort in a bowl.

1. Heat a large saucepan over a medium–high heat.

2. Add the bacon and cook until golden, then remove and set aside.

3. Add the butter to the pan and, once melted, add the onions, carrots and celery and fry for a couple of minutes until softened.

4. Add the garlic and red pepper and fry for another minute.

5. Add the potatoes and stock, bring to the boil, then simmer for 15 minutes.

6. Whisk together the milk and cornflour and add to the pan along with the cooked chicken and the sweetcorn. Simmer until the soup thickens (approx. 8 minutes).

7. Taste and season with salt and freshly ground black pepper, and serve each bowl with a sprinkle of fresh chives and cooked bacon.

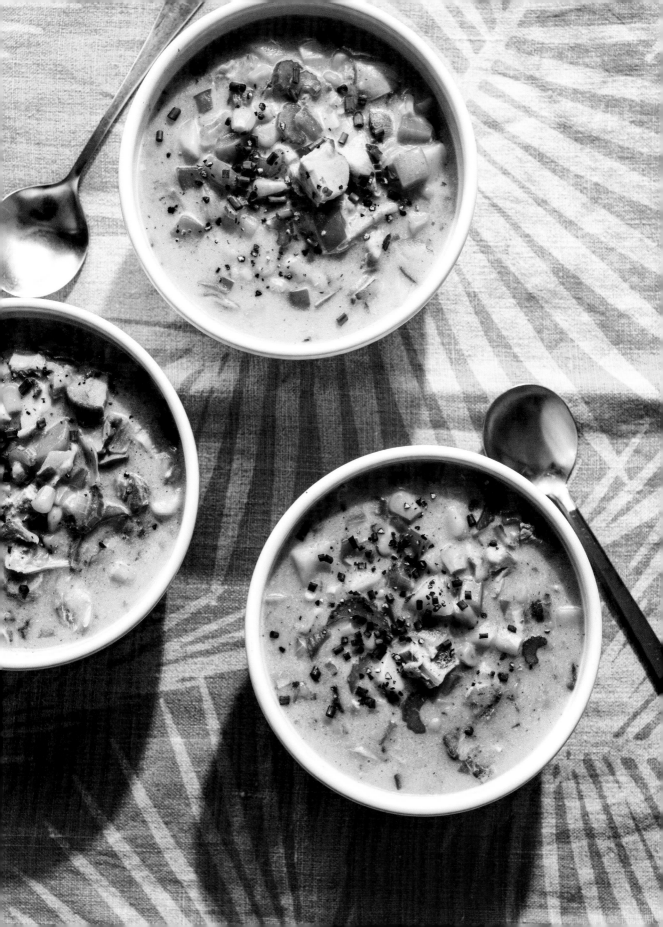

254
Calories

DF

Ham, Vegetable and Pearl Barley Soup

KCALS
254

FAT
3.7g

SAT FAT
1.2g

CARBS
33.1g

SUGARS
6.2g

FIBRE
4.6g

PROTEIN
19.8g

SALT
2.96g

SERVES 6

olive oil spray
1 onion, finely diced
200g (7oz) carrots, diced
200g (7oz) celery, diced
200g (7oz) potatoes,
    peeled and diced
200g (7oz) butternut
    squash, peeled and diced
2 teaspoons dried
    mixed (Italian) herbs
150g (5½oz) pearl barley
1.9 litres (3¼ pints) chicken
    or ham stock
2 bay leaves
250g (9oz) cooked ham (or
    bacon), chopped
salt and freshly ground
    black pepper
2–3 tablespoons chopped
    fresh parsley

We are a family that loves soups, and they are a great way to get vegetables into even the fussiest of children (or adults). My children often avoid certain vegetables if they're just served on a plate, but if they are in a soup they will devour the whole lot. This ham, vegetable and pearl barley soup is hearty and makes a complete meal in a bowl.

1. Place a deep saucepan over a medium high heat and spray with the olive oil.

2. Add the onion, carrots and celery and fry until softened.

3. Add the potatoes, butternut squash and mixed herbs and stir to combine.

4. Add the pearl barley, stock, bay leaves and ham, bring to the boil, then cover and simmer for 30 minutes until the barley is cooked.

5. Taste and season with salt and freshly ground black pepper.

6. Stir in the chopped fresh parsley.

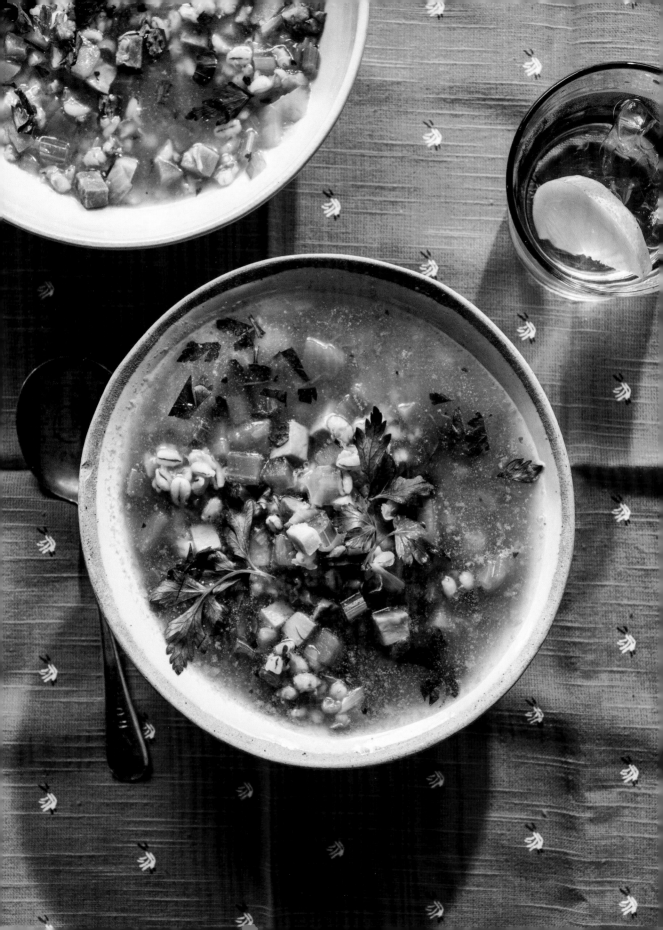

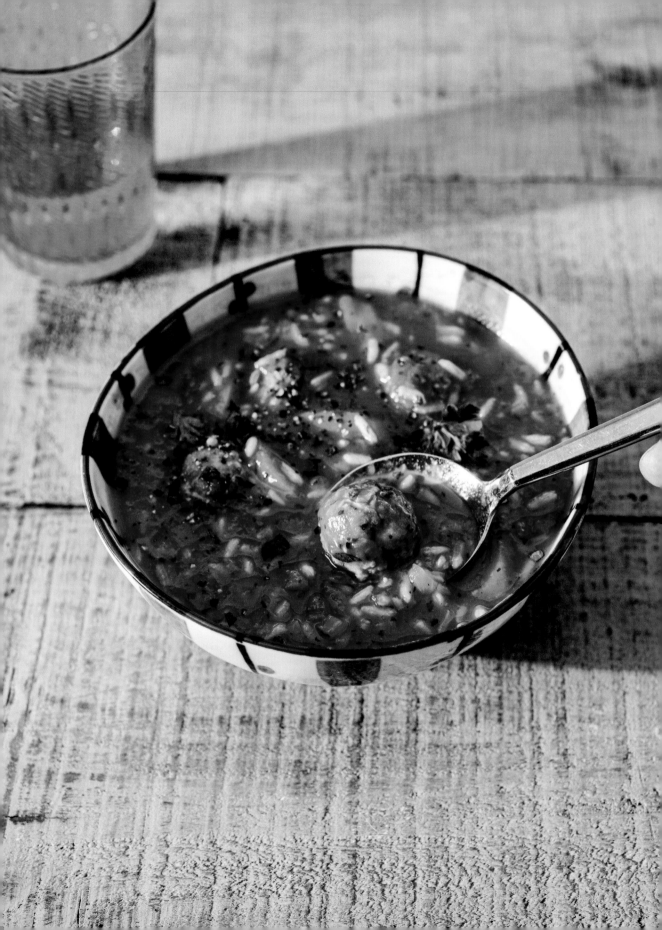

Spicy Turkey Meatballs and Rice Soup

251 Calories

GF

SERVES 6

For the meatballs:
100g (3½oz) courgettes (zucchini)
400g (14oz) extra lean (5% fat) turkey mince
30g (1oz) Parmesan, grated
1 teaspoon dried oregano
½ teaspoon garlic powder
½ teaspoon salt
pinch of freshly ground black pepper

For the soup:
olive oil spray
1 onion, finely diced
2 garlic cloves, crushed
1 large carrot, halved and thinly sliced
½ teaspoon fennel seeds, crushed in a pestle and mortar
pinch of red chilli flakes
2 teaspoons dried mixed (Italian) herbs
2 tablespoons tomato purée (paste)
1.2 litres (2 pints) chicken stock
400g (14oz) tin of chopped tomatoes
180g (6oz) passata
100g (3½oz) long-grain rice
salt and freshly ground black pepper
chopped fresh parsley

This makes for such a fantastic and filling lunch or dinner, these cheesy turkey meatballs and rice in a flavorsome spicy tomato broth are delicately flavoured with fennel and herbs.

1. Preheat the oven to 180°C/160°C fan/350°F/gas 4 and line a baking tray with parchment paper.

2. Grate the courgettes and squeeze out excess moisture, then put them into a bowl with the turkey mince, Parmesan, oregano, garlic powder, salt and freshly ground black pepper.

3. Roll the mixture into 30 small meatballs and place them on the lined baking tray.

4. Bake in the oven for 12–15 minutes, until lightly golden, then remove and set aside.

5. Place a large deep saucepan on a medium heat and spray with olive oil, then add the onion, garlic and carrot and fry for a couple of minutes.

6. Add the fennel seeds, chilli flakes, mixed herbs and tomato purée and stir to coat the vegetables.

7. Pour in the stock, tinned tomatoes and passata and add the meatballs.

8. Bring to the boil, simmer for 10 minutes, then add the rice and simmer until it is cooked.

9. Taste and season with salt and freshly ground black pepper, and sprinkle with chopped parsley to serve.

KCALS
251

FAT
6.2g

SAT FAT
2.4g

CARBS
22.0g

SUGARS
7.3g

FIBRE
3.4g

PROTEIN
25.4g

SALT
1.83g

Chicken Dill Pickle Salad

SERVES 2

For the croutons:
60g (2oz) wholemeal
  (whole wheat) bread,
  cut into cubes
olive oil spray
¼ teaspoon garlic powder
¼ teaspoon onion powder
1 teaspoon dried dill
pinch of dried mixed (Italian)
  herbs
salt and freshly ground
  black pepper

For the chicken:
½ teaspoon salt
½ teaspoon dried parsley
¼ teaspoon dried thyme
½ teaspoon paprika
250g (9oz) boneless skinless
  chicken breasts, flattened
cooking oil spray

For the salad:
1 head of romaine lettuce
½ cucumber
80g (3oz) dill pickles, diced
3 spring onions (scallions),
  chopped
80g (3oz) fat-free Greek
  yoghurt
3 tablespoons light
  mayonnaise
3 tablespoons dill pickle juice
  (vinegar)
1 teaspoon chopped fresh dill
¼ teaspoon garlic powder
¼ teaspoon onion powder
1 teaspoon dried parsley
salt and freshly ground
  black pepper

This ultimate salad is inspired by a beautiful meal I once had at one of my favourite places to eat at home in Canada. The flavour from the dill pickles takes it to a whole new level.

1. Preheat the oven to 200°C/180°C fan/400°F/gas 6.

2. First, prepare the croutons. Put the bread into a bowl, spray with the olive oil, add the garlic powder, onion powder, dill, mixed herbs and a pinch of salt and freshly ground black pepper, and toss to coat. Spread on a baking tray lined with parchment paper and bake for approx. 8–10 minutes, until golden and crispy.

3. Meanwhile, mix the salt, parsley, thyme and paprika together in a small bowl and rub into the chicken. Place a frying pan over a medium–high heat and spray with the oil. Add the chicken and brown (approx. 3–4 minutes), then flip and cook the other side. Remove and set aside while you prepare the rest of the salad.

4. Put the romaine lettuce, cucumber, pickles and spring onions into a bowl for the salad.

5. Mix together the yoghurt, mayonnaise, pickle juice, fresh dill, garlic powder, onion powder and dried parsley to make a dressing. Season with salt and freshly ground black pepper.

6. Add the dressing to the bowl of salad and toss to coat.

7. Using a sharp knife, slice up the chicken. Add it to the salad and sprinkle over the croutons.

8. Serve and enjoy!

Optional:
Crumble in some feta cheese.

Tip:
Make a triple batch of the dressing –
it's perfect on any salad.

KCALS	**406**
FAT	**14g**
SAT FAT	**0.9g**
CARBS	**21.5g**
SUGARS	**9.1g**
FIBRE	**10.8g**
PROTEIN	**43.1g**
SALT	**2.59g**

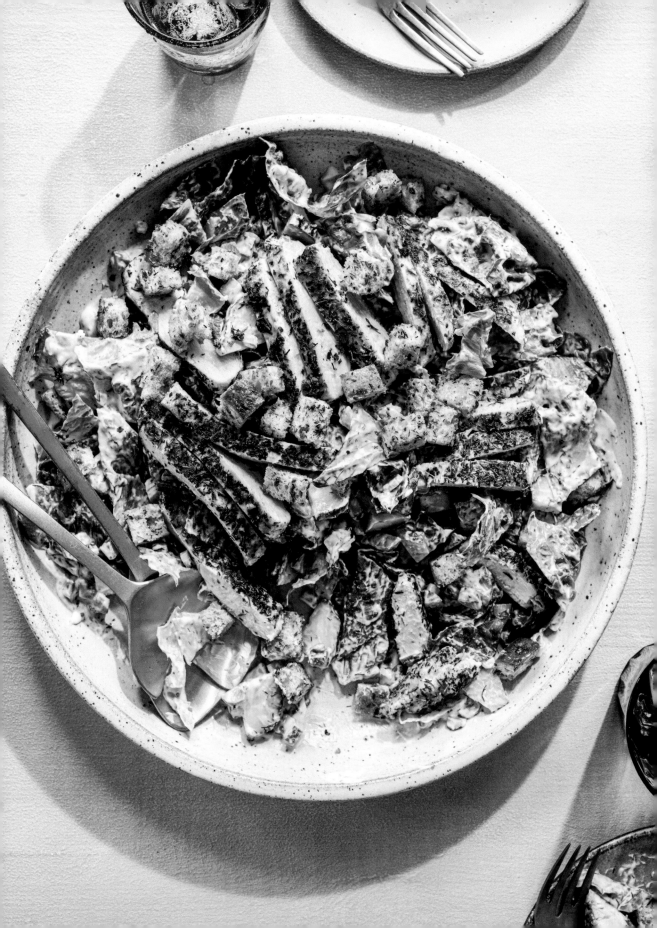

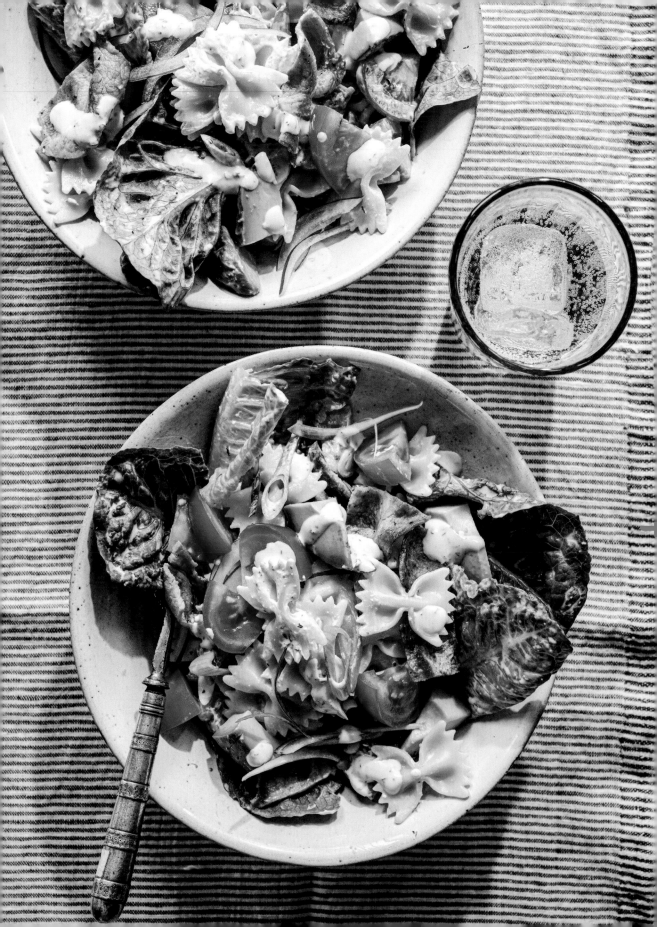

BLT Pasta Salad

SERVES 4

180g (6oz) fusilli pasta
(or other pasta of your
choice)
200g (7oz) romaine lettuce,
chopped
250g (9oz) ripe tomatoes,
diced
60g (2oz) red onion,
finely diced
3 spring onions (scallions),
sliced
100g (3½oz) diced avocado
8 slices of lean smoked back
bacon (fat removed),
cooked and chopped

For the dressing:
180g (6oz) plain fat-free
yoghurt
2 tablespoons light
mayonnaise
2 tablespoons light soured
cream
1 teaspoon Worcestershire
sauce
1 teaspoon garlic powder
1 teaspoon onion powder
2 teaspoons dried chives
2 teaspoons dried parsley
1 teaspoon sweetener
salt and freshly ground
black pepper

Gluten-free:
Use gluten-free pasta.

Optional:
Add some grated or cubed
Cheddar.

Tip:
Use this dressing for any
salad.

**All the best components of an amazing BLT sandwich in
a tasty pasta salad that is perfect for lunches, picnics
and barbecues.**

1. Cook the pasta in a pan of boiling salted water until al dente,
then drain and set aside to cool.

2. Put the cooked pasta into a large bowl and add the lettuce,
tomatoes, red onion, spring onions, avocado and bacon. Toss
well to combine.

3. Mix the dressing ingredients together in a bowl, then drizzle
over the salad.

4. Taste and season with salt and freshly ground black pepper.

KCALS	**422**
FAT	**17.8g**
SAT FAT	**5.2g**
CARBS	**42.4g**
SUGARS	**8.7g**
FIBRE	**6.1g**
PROTEIN	**19.8g**
SALT	**1.55g**

Tuna Niçoise Salad

KCALS
295

FAT
10.3g

SAT FAT
2.3g

CARBS
21.7g

SUGARS
7.4g

FIBRE
7.8g

PROTEIN
24.9g

SALT
1.84g

SERVES 4

4 large eggs
400g (14oz) baby potatoes,
    halved
450ml (16fl oz) chicken stock
olive oil spray
1 garlic clove, crushed
400g (14oz) French green
    beans
80g (3oz) frozen sweetcorn
2 x 145g (5¼oz) tins of flaked
    tuna in water, drained
2 ripe tomatoes, quartered
80g (3oz) butterhead or
    romaine lettuce
12 black Kalamata olives,
    pitted
salt and freshly ground
    black pepper

For the dressing:
1 tablespoon extra virgin
    olive oil
2 tablespoons fresh
    lemon juice
½ tablespoon Dijon mustard
1 teaspoon honey
½ teaspoon finely chopped
    fresh basil
½ teaspoon finely chopped
    fresh thyme
¼ teaspoon garlic powder
¼ teaspoon onion powder
pinch of salt

Tip:
You can use this simple
dressing for any salad of
your choice.

There really are no rules when it comes to a Niçoise salad: I love
to serve mine with warm baby potatoes, green beans, sweetcorn
and perfect soft-boiled eggs. All finished off with a simple light
Dijon mustard dressing.

1. Whisk together the ingredients for the dressing and set aside to
let the flavours combine.

2. Put the eggs into a small saucepan of boiling water over a medium
heat, cover and continue to bubble for 6 minutes, then drain and
put the eggs into an ice bath. Once cool, carefully peel.

3. Put the potatoes into a saucepan and cover with the stock. Bring
to the boil, then lower the heat, cover and simmer for approx.
10–12 minutes, until tender.

4. Drain the potatoes, reserving 125ml (4fl oz) of the stock. Set aside.

5. Place a frying pan on a medium heat and spray with olive oil.
Add the garlic and sauté until lightly golden, then add the green
beans and the sweetcorn and toss to coat. Pour in the reserved
stock and reduce down around the beans until cooked.

6. Add the potatoes, spray with a little cooking oil, and toss in the
pan, just enough to warm up the potatoes with the beans and corn.
Serve plated with the tuna, tomatoes, lettuce and olives, then slice
the eggs in half and add those too. Season everything with salt and
freshly ground black pepper.

7. Drizzle with the dressing and enjoy.

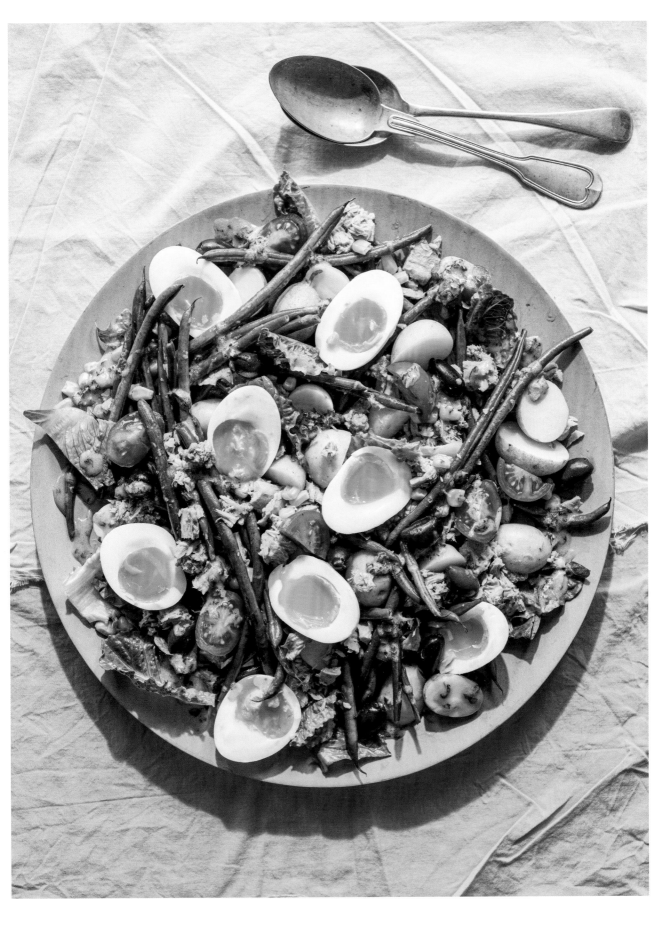

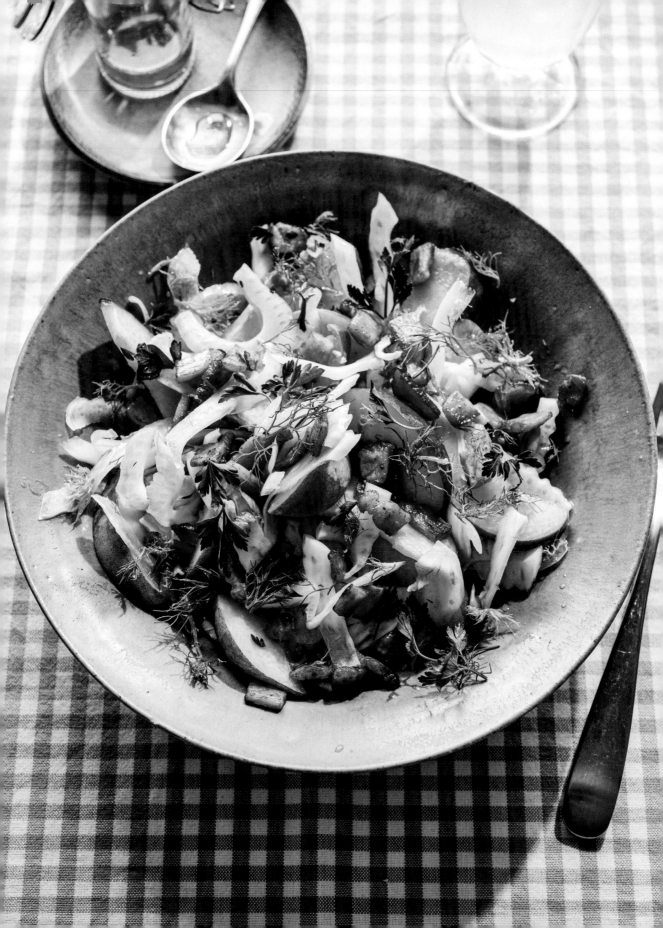

Bacon, Peach and Fennel Salad

SERVES 2

cooking oil spray
4 slices of lean smoked
  bacon (fat removed), diced
1 large fennel bulb, trimmed
  and thinly sliced (reserve
  the fronds)
3 ripe peaches
1 tablespoon extra virgin
  olive oil
1 tablespoon red wine vinegar
a few fresh parsley leaves
salt and freshly ground
  black pepper

This salad is a flavour explosion on the palate, delicious as a light lunch or served as a side to a main course. Crunchy fennel, sweet ripened peaches and cooked smoky bacon, all finished off with a red wine vinegar and olive oil dressing.

1. Put a frying pan on a medium heat and spray it with cooking oil. Add the bacon and cook until golden, then set aside.

2. Slice the fennel thinly, using a sharp knife or a mandolin. Put into a bowl.

3. Slice the peaches in half, remove the stones, then slice each peach half into 6 wedges.

4. Whisk the olive oil with the vinegar, drizzle over the fennel and toss to coat.

5. Top with the peaches, scatter over the cooked bacon, and add a few fresh parsley leaves and fennel fronds.

6. Season with salt and freshly ground black pepper.

7. Enjoy as a light meal or a side to a main meal of your choice. (It's especially great with a grilled seasoned chicken breast.)

KCALS
252

FAT
14.8g

SAT FAT
4.1g

CARBS
14.1g

SUGARS
13.9g

FIBRE
7.2g

PROTEIN
12.2g

SALT
1.43g

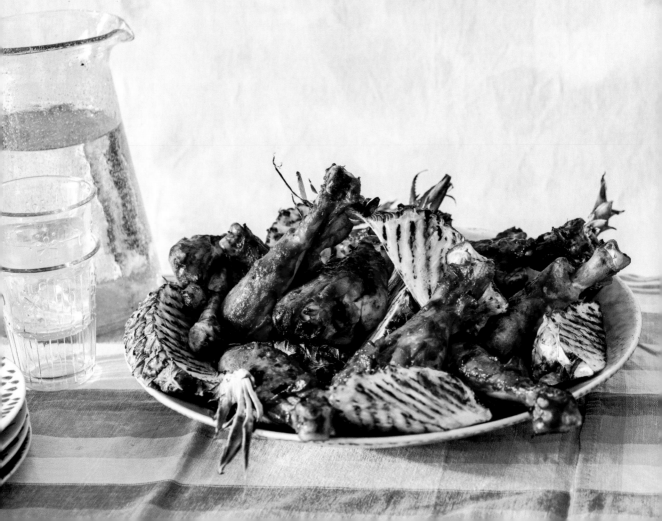

Poultry

Creamy Cajun Chicken

One-pot Chicken,
Tomato and Fennel Orzo

Chicken Ramen

Hunter's Chicken
Meatloaf

Garlic Mayo Chicken
Traybake

Braised Chicken
Casserole

Healthier Chicken
Pot Pie

Huli Huli Chicken
with Spicy Grilled
Pineapple

One-pot Firecracker
Chicken Rice

Butter Chicken
Lasagne

Creamy Red Pepper
Penne with Chicken

Umami Chicken
Traybake

Chicken Greek
Gyro Bowls

Chilli Lime Chicken
and Rice Bake

Orange Chicken

Creamy Cajun Chicken

GF

KCALS
364

FAT
11.4g

SAT FAT
2.4g

CARBS
6.3g

SUGARS
4.9g

FIBRE
3.5g

PROTEIN
57.3g

SALT
1.17g

SERVES 4

4 skinless chicken breasts
    (approx. 200g/7oz each),
    flattened
olive oil spray
4 garlic cloves, crushed
1 red pepper, diced
1 green pepper, diced
1 tablespoon tomato purée
    (paste)
420ml (¾ pint) chicken
    stock
120g (4oz) light cream
    cheese
30g (1oz) Parmesan, grated
salt and freshly ground
    black pepper
chopped fresh parsley

For the Cajun seasoning:
1 tablespoon paprika
1 teaspoon onion powder
1 teaspoon garlic powder
½ teaspoon dried oregano
½ teaspoon dried thyme
¼–½ teaspoon cayenne

Swap:
If you don't like peppers
you can try swapping them
out for other vegetables
– mushrooms, spinach,
courgettes (zucchini) all
work well.

Sides suggestions:
Pair with rice, potatoes, pasta
or for a low-carb option
some cauliflower rice (see
page 239) or steamed/
roasted veggies.

**A wonderful dinner that is ready and on the table in less than
30 minutes – this tender chicken with peppers in a creamy Cajun
sauce pairs really well with a variety of sides.**

1. Mix all the Cajun seasoning ingredients together in a bowl.
Rub half the seasoning into the chicken breasts.

2. Place a frying pan over a medium–high heat and spray with olive
oil. Add the chicken breasts and brown on both sides (approx.
5 minutes each side), then remove from the pan and set aside.

3. Add the garlic and peppers to the pan and fry for a couple of minutes.

4. Add the rest of the Cajun seasoning, the tomato purée, stock
and cream cheese, and stir until the cheese has melted.

5. Put the chicken back into the pan and simmer until it is cooked
through and the sauce has thickened.

6. Add the Parmesan and stir until melted. Taste and season as
needed with salt and freshly ground black pepper.

7. Sprinkle with chopped fresh parsley.

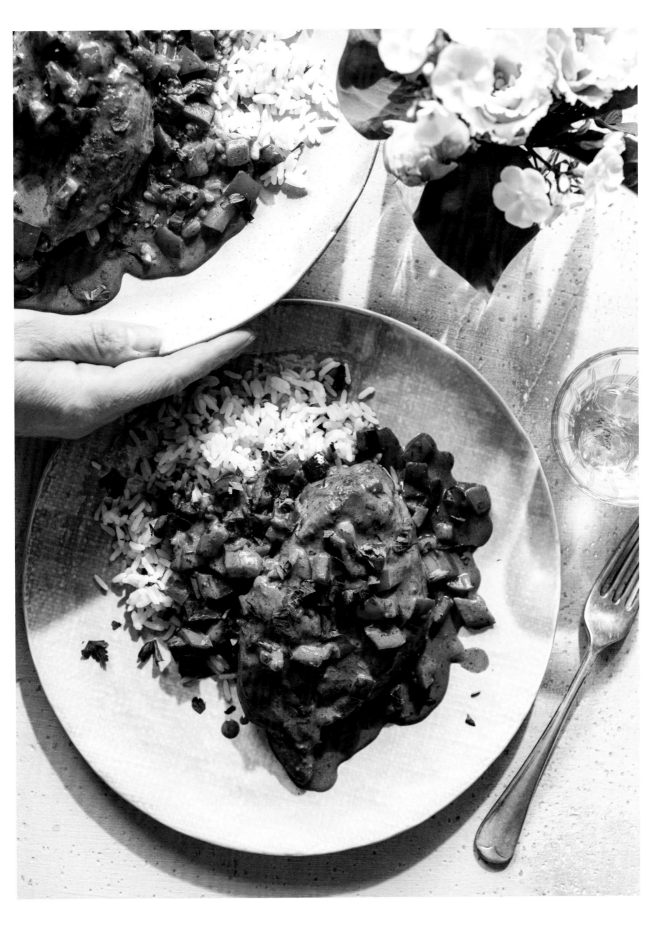

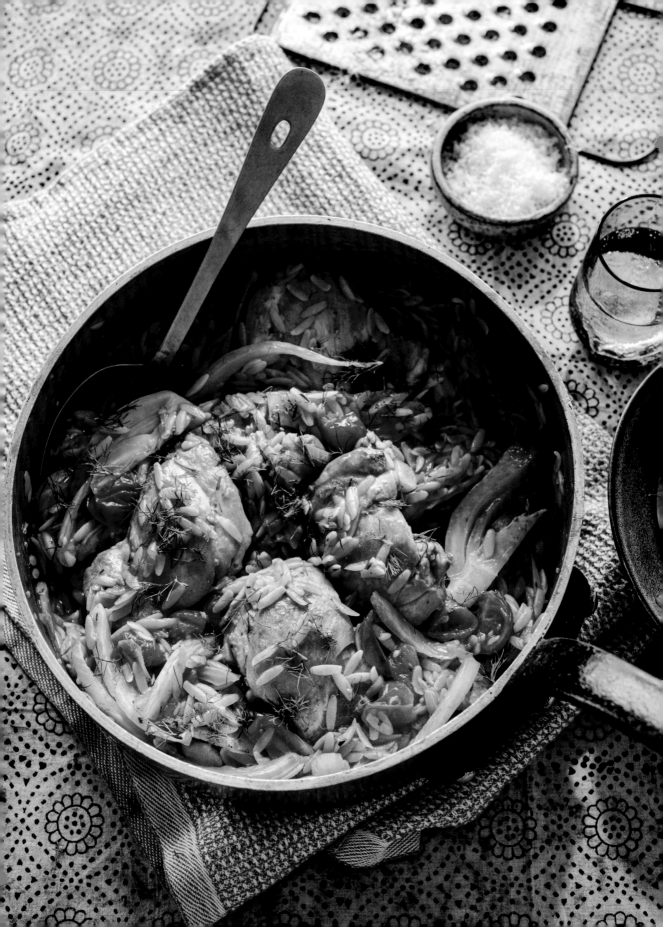

One-pot Chicken, Tomato and Fennel Orzo

478 Calories

DF

SERVES 4

600g (1lb 5oz) boneless skinless chicken thighs, trimmed of any visible fat
salt and freshly ground black pepper
olive oil spray
1 tablespoon olive oil
1 fennel bulb, chopped (reserve the fronds)
300g (10½oz) cherry or grape tomatoes, halved
2 garlic cloves, crushed
1 teaspoon dried oregano
1 tablespoon white wine vinegar
1 tablespoon tomato purée (paste)
200g (7oz) dried orzo pasta
720ml (1¼ pints) chicken stock
grated Parmesan (optional)

Dairy-free:
Omit the optional cheese.

Fennel is such a versatile vegetable and has an amazing flavour, especially when paired with tomatoes, as in this one-pot recipe with chicken and orzo. An effortless meal that is a life-saver for any weeknight.

1. Season the chicken on both sides with salt and freshly ground black pepper.

2. Place a deep non-stick frying pan over a medium–high heat and spray with olive oil spray.

3. Add the chicken and cook until golden, then flip and cook the other side. Remove from the pan and set aside.

4. Add the olive oil to the pan, then add the fennel and cook until lightly golden and slightly softened.

5. Add the tomatoes and garlic and continue to cook until the tomatoes start to soften.

6. Add the oregano, vinegar, tomato purée and orzo and stir to combine.

7. Pour in the stock, then place the chicken thighs on top.

8. Bring to the boil, then reduce the heat, cover the pan and simmer for 12–15 minutes, until the stock is absorbed and the orzo is cooked.

9. Taste and season with salt and freshly ground black pepper as needed, and serve garnished with the reserved fennel fronds and with grated Parmesan, if you like.

KCALS
478

FAT
14.3g

SAT FAT
3.6g

CARBS
42.3g

SUGARS
5.1g

FIBRE
5.6g

PROTEIN
42.1g

SALT
1.16g

Chicken Ramen

DF

KCALS
459

FAT
8.8g

SAT FAT
2.3g

CARBS
43.3g

SUGARS
9.9g

FIBRE
6.6g

PROTEIN
48.3g

SALT
5.06g

SERVES 2

1 boneless skinless chicken breast (approx. 200g/7oz), flattened
½ teaspoon garlic powder
½ teaspoon onion powder
salt and freshly ground black pepper
cooking oil spray
2 eggs
5 spring onions (scallions), sliced
1 carrot, grated or julienned
50g (2oz) mushrooms, sliced (shiitake mushrooms give the best flavour, but any mushrooms are fine)
½ tablespoon grated fresh ginger
2 garlic cloves, crushed
240ml (9fl oz) chicken stock
2 tablespoons soy sauce
½ tablespoon fish sauce
1 tablespoon mirin (or dry sherry)
1 bok choy
80g (3oz) dried egg noodles (or low-fat dried ramen noodles)

Optional:
Add a final drizzle of sriracha or a sprinkling of red chilli flakes for a spicy kick.

Note:
If you don't have any mirin or sherry, you can use a pinch of sweetener.

Reducing salt:
To reduce the salt content, use low-sodium soy sauce and stock.

My family are big on ramen, but some of the ramen noodles that come with those little seasoning packs can have a whole load of calories and not contain the healthiest of ingredients. So I often make up these quick chicken ramen bowls instead. Traditionally making ramen broth is a long process, achieving that full flavour by making the broth completely from scratch, but when you want an easy meal this simple version is just the ticket.

1. Season the chicken breast with the garlic powder, onion powder and a pinch of salt and freshly ground black pepper.

2. Place a frying pan over a medium–high heat and spray with cooking oil. Add the chicken and cook on one side for approx. 5 minutes, until golden, then flip and repeat on the other side. Remove and set aside.

3. Bring a saucepan of water to the boil. Add the eggs and allow to bubble for 6 minutes, then remove them to an ice bath.

4. Place a large saucepan on a medium heat and spray with cooking oil. Add half the spring onions and carrots, and all the mushrooms, ginger and garlic, and fry for a couple of minutes.

5. Add the stock, soy sauce, fish sauce and mirin.

6. Bring to the boil, then simmer, covered, for 20 minutes. Drop in the bok choy for the last couple of minutes.

7. While the broth is cooking, peel the eggs.

8. Cook the noodles according to the package instructions.

9. Once the stock is ready you can build your ramen.

10. Slice the cooked chicken and add some to each of your bowls with the noodles.

11. Ladle in the stock (with the veggies), ensuring you add half a bok choy to each bowl. Top with the reserved spring onions and carrots, then slice the eggs in half and add to the bowls.

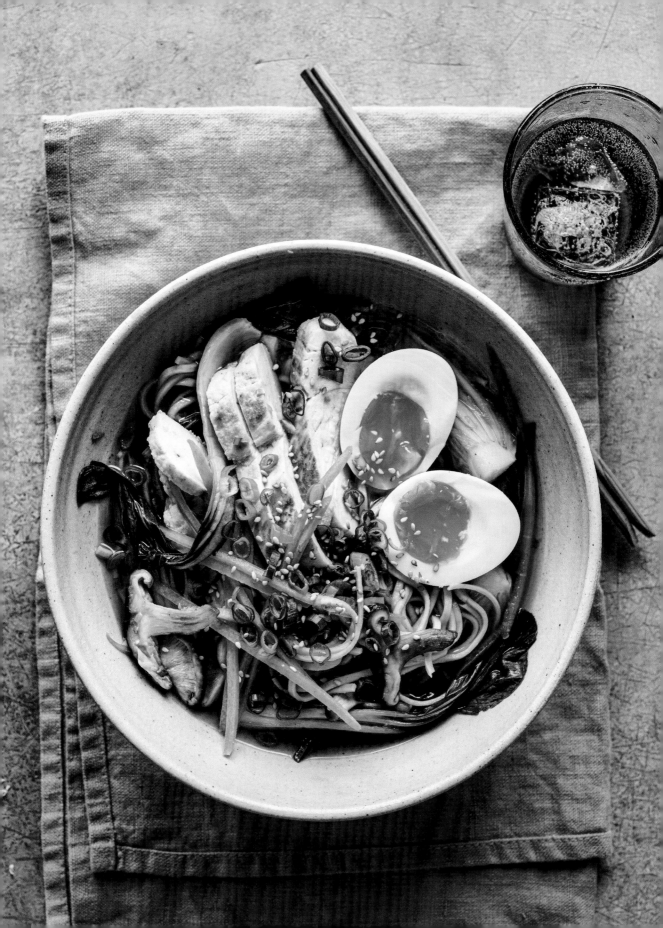

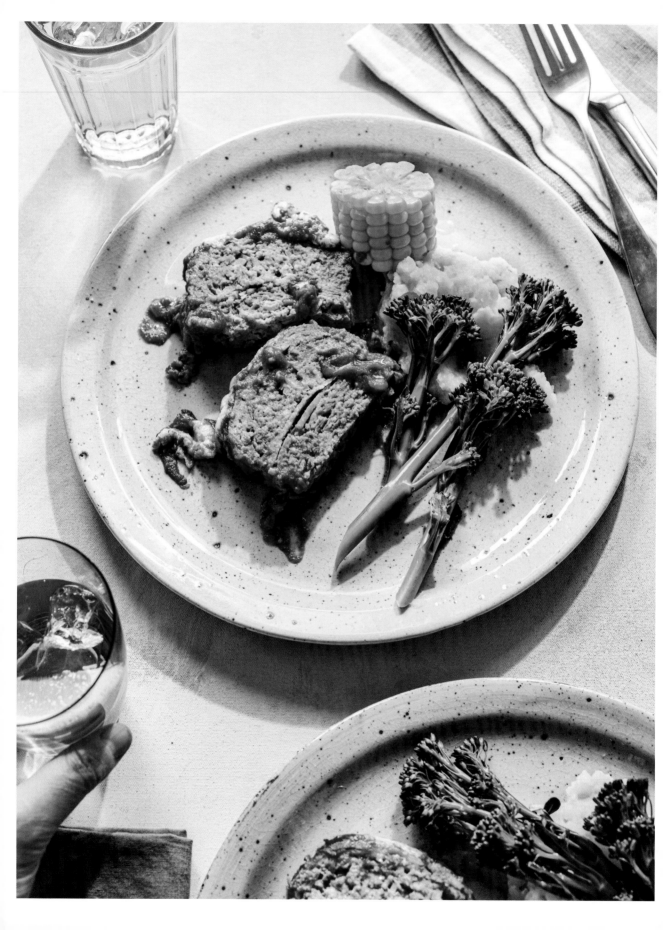

Hunter's Chicken Meatloaf

SERVES 4

For the barbecue sauce:
180ml (6oz) passata
3 tablespoons tomato purée
 (paste)
2 tablespoons balsamic
 vinegar
2 tablespoons maple syrup
2 teaspoons paprika
½ tablespoon Worcestershire
 sauce
½ teaspoon smoked paprika
2 teaspoons yellow American
 mustard

For the meatloaf:
olive oil spray
1 small onion, diced
500g (1lb 2oz) extra lean
 (5% fat) chicken mince
 (you can use turkey mince)
1 large egg
30g (1oz) fine dried
 breadcrumbs
¼ teaspoon onion powder
¼ teaspoon garlic powder
1 teaspoon paprika
8 slices of lean smoked
 bacon (fat removed),
 chopped
40g (1½oz) Red Leicester or
 Cheddar, grated
40g (1½oz) mozzarella,
 grated
chopped fresh parsley

Low-carb side suggestion:
Swap mashed potatoes
for cauliflower, butternut
squash, celeriac (celery root)
or swede mash.

Freezing:
To reheat after freezing,
defrost in the fridge then
warm through in an oven
preheated to 180°C/160°C
fan/350°F/gas 4.

If you thought you loved regular Hunter's chicken, wait until you try this amazing Hunter's chicken meatloaf, which is one of my family's favourite recipes. This show-stopping meatloaf with layers of smoky bacon is finished off with an easy barbecue sauce and melted cheese.

1. Preheat the oven to 180°C/160°C fan/350°F/gas 4.

2. Place a frying pan over a medium–high heat and spray with olive oil. Add the onion and fry until lightly browned and softened.

3. Remove the onion from the pan and put it into a bowl with the chicken mince, egg, breadcrumbs, onion powder, garlic powder and paprika, and mix to combine.

4. Place half the meatloaf mixture in a large loaf tin, pushing it down tightly, then layer with half the bacon, add the remaining meatloaf mixture and top with the remaining bacon. Run a spatula around the sides to create a space (this is so the sauce can cover all the meatloaf). If you don't have a loaf tin, you can form the mixture into a free-standing loaf on a small rimmed baking tray.

5. Combine the sauce ingredients in a bowl and pour over the top of the meatloaf.

6. Bake in the oven for 40 minutes, then top with the cheese and put back into the oven for 10–15 minutes, until the cheese is melted.

7. Sprinkle with chopped fresh parsley, and allow to rest for 10 minutes before slicing.

8. Slice and serve with your choice of sides. Mashed potatoes with steamed green vegetables and sweetcorn are our favourites.

448
Calories

KCALS
448

FAT
21.5g

SAT FAT
8.5g

CARBS
23.1g

SUGARS
13.0g

FIBRE
2.4g

PROTEIN
39.3g

SALT
3.57g

Garlic Mayo Chicken Traybake

SERVES 4

cooking oil spray
600g (1lb 5oz) waxy
    potatoes, diced
4 skinless chicken breasts
    (200g/7oz each), flattened
2 teaspoons paprika
1 teaspoon dried mixed
    (Italian) herbs
¼ teaspoon onion powder
salt and freshly ground
    black pepper
400g (14oz) courgettes
    (zucchini), sliced

For the mayo topping:
6 tablespoons light
    mayonnaise
4 garlic cloves, crushed
1 teaspoon dried parsley
20g (¾oz) Parmesan, grated
pinch of freshly ground
    black pepper

Gluten-free:
Use gluten-free mayonnaise.

Low-carb swap:
Swap the potato for cubes
of butternut squash.

KCALS	**450**
FAT	**15.0g**
SAT FAT	**3.5g**
CARBS	**26.0g**
SUGARS	**4.2g**
FIBRE	**4.7g**
PROTEIN	**50.5g**
SALT	**1.50g**

A cook-in-one-pan meal that packs heaps of flavour. Juicy, garlicky mayo-and-Parmesan-topped chicken breasts, with golden baked potatoes and courgette (zucchini) slices.

1. Preheat the oven to 220°C/200°C fan/425°F/gas 7. Line a large baking tray with parchment paper and spray with cooking oil.

2. Make the mayo topping. In a bowl, combine the mayo, garlic, parsley, Parmesan and a pinch of freshly ground black pepper. Set aside.

3. Spread out the potatoes on the lined tray, spray with cooking oil and season with salt. Place in the oven and bake for 35 minutes.

4. Place the chicken breasts in between 2 sheets of parchment paper or cling film and flatten with a rolling pin or meat tenderizer. Mix together the paprika, herbs, 1 teaspoon of salt, onion powder and a pinch of freshly ground black pepper in a bowl and rub this spice mix into the chicken breasts. Transfer to a large plate.

5. Top each breast with the mayo topping.

6. Once the potatoes have baked for 35 minutes, remove the tray from the oven and push the potatoes over so they take up one third of the tray.

7. Carefully add the chicken pieces to the next third, and add the courgettes to the final third. Season the courgettes with a little salt and freshly ground black pepper and spray with cooking oil.

8. Put the traybake back into the oven for a further 20–25 minutes, until the chicken is cooked through.

9. Serve and enjoy!

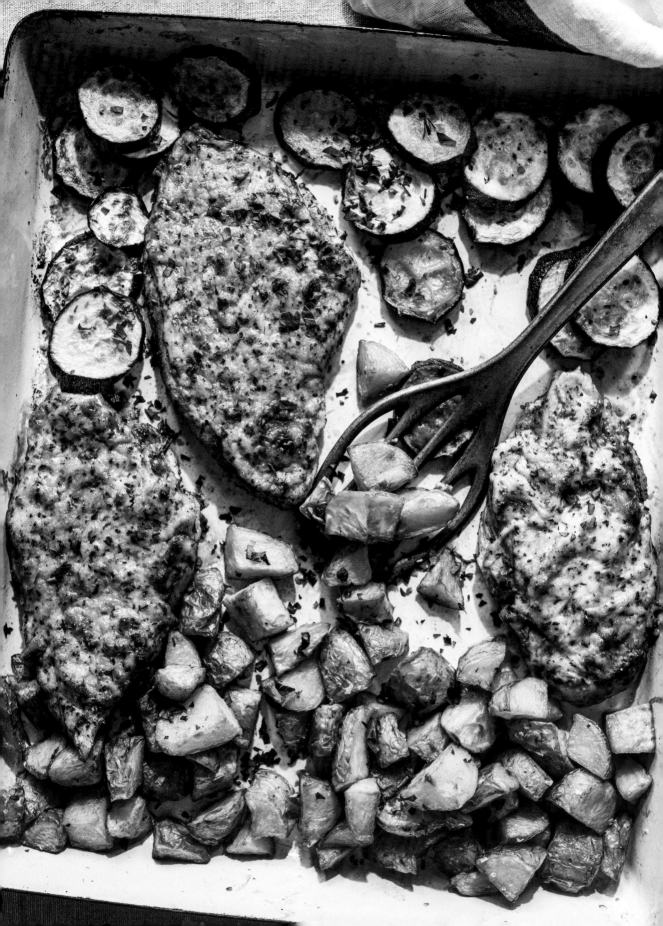

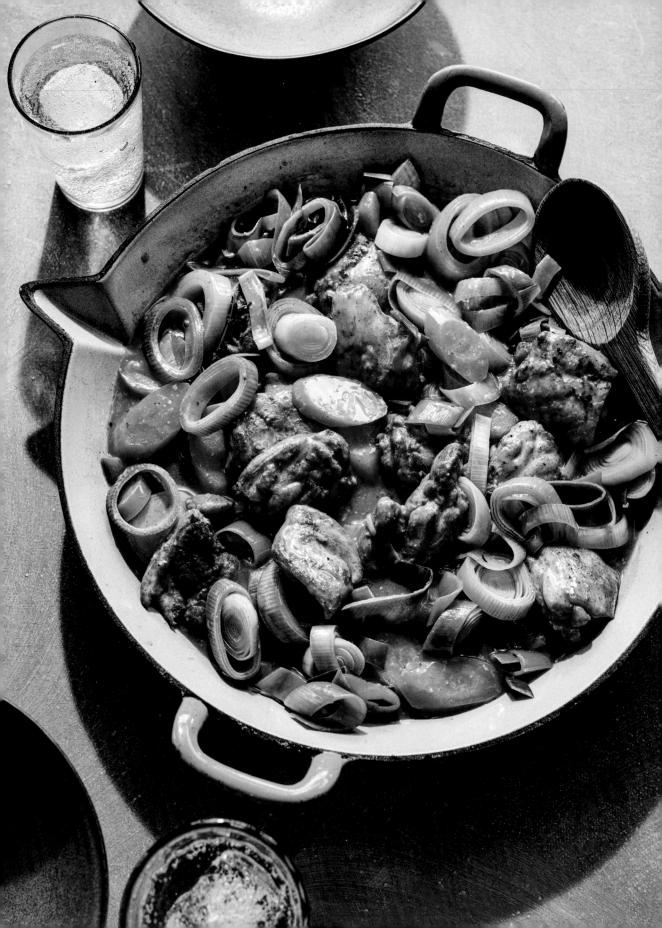

Braised Chicken Casserole

SERVES 4

olive oil spray
500g (1lb 2oz) boneless
  skinless chicken thighs,
  halved
1 teaspoon paprika
salt and freshly ground
  black pepper
2 leeks, thinly sliced and
  rinsed (remove tough
  outer leaves)
3 garlic cloves, crushed
2 carrots, halved
  lengthways and cut into
  2.5cm (1 inch) pieces
1 tablespoon chopped fresh
  thyme
1 bay leaf
2 tablespoons white wine
  vinegar
575ml (20fl oz) chicken
  stock
1 tablespoon cornflour
  (cornstarch)

Side suggestions:
Mash (for example, the
rustic kale, leek and potato
mash on page 255) or roast
potatoes. Sweet potato mash
is also delicious with this.

Lower-carb option:
Cauliflower mash, celeriac
mash or roasted seasoned
butternut squash cubes.

Freezing:
To reheat after freezing,
simply defrost in the fridge,
then warm through in the
microwave or in a saucepan
over a medium heat.

Succulent, tender chicken thighs, braised in a flavoursome broth with vegetables for a comforting any-day-of-the-week meal that the whole family will love.

1. Place a frying pan over a medium–high heat and spray with olive oil.

2. Season the halved chicken thighs with the paprika and a pinch of salt and freshly ground black pepper, fry until golden on each side, then remove and set aside.

3. Spray the pan again, then add the leeks and garlic and fry until softened.

4. Return the chicken to the pan along with the carrots, thyme, bay leaf, vinegar and stock. Bring to the boil, then cover and simmer for 25–30 minutes.

5. Mix the cornflour with a little water to make a slurry. Add this to the pan and simmer until the sauce thickens (5–8 minutes).

6. Taste and season with salt and freshly ground black pepper.

KCALS	**248**
FAT	**9.5g**
SAT FAT	**2.6g**
CARBS	**9.4g**
SUGARS	**4.6g**
FIBRE	**4.3g**
PROTEIN	**29.1g**
SALT	**0.98g**

Healthier Chicken Pot Pie

SERVES 4

olive oil spray
350g (12½oz) skinless
  chicken breast (or a mix of
  thigh and breast meat)
½ teaspoon dried thyme
salt and freshly ground
  black pepper
1 tablespoon butter
1 onion, diced
150g (5½oz) carrots,
  cut into small cubes
1 stalk of celery, chopped
240ml (9fl oz) chicken stock
60g (2oz) frozen sweetcorn
60g (2oz) frozen peas
240ml (9fl oz) milk
1½ tablespoons cornflour
  (cornstarch)
4 sheets of filo pastry
1 egg, beaten

Freezing:
You could freeze the filling
to use later.

When it comes to pies, we often feel we need to avoid them because pastry can be quite high in calories. This healthier made-from-scratch chicken pot pie has all the mouthwatering components you'd expect, including a creamy-style sauce, and is finished off with a light golden filo pastry topping.

1. Place a saucepan on a medium–high heat and spray with olive oil. Add the chicken, season with the thyme, salt and freshly ground black pepper, fry until lightly golden, then remove from the pan and set aside.

2. Add the butter to the pan. Once melted, add the onion, carrots and celery and fry until the onion is translucent. Pour in the stock and simmer for about 10 minutes. Put the chicken back into the pan and add the sweetcorn, peas and milk.

3. Mix the cornflour (cornstarch) with a little water to make a slurry and add this to the pan, simmering until the sauce thickens (about 5–8 minutes). Taste the sauce and adjust the seasoning with salt and freshly ground black pepper if needed.

4. Preheat the oven to 200°C/180°C fan/ 400°F/gas 6.

5. Transfer the mixture to a 23cm (9in) round oven dish and allow to cool slightly. Break each sheet of filo in half, then squash each half into a rough ball and place these on top of the chicken mixture, repeating with the rest of pastry until the pie is all covered.

6. Brush over the top with the beaten egg and spray with a little olive oil.

7. Bake in the oven at for about 25 minutes, or until lightly golden on top.

KCALS
384

FAT
11.3g

SAT FAT
3.9g

CARBS
37.2g

SUGARS
9.5g

FIBRE
5.2g

PROTEIN
30.7g

SALT
1.01g

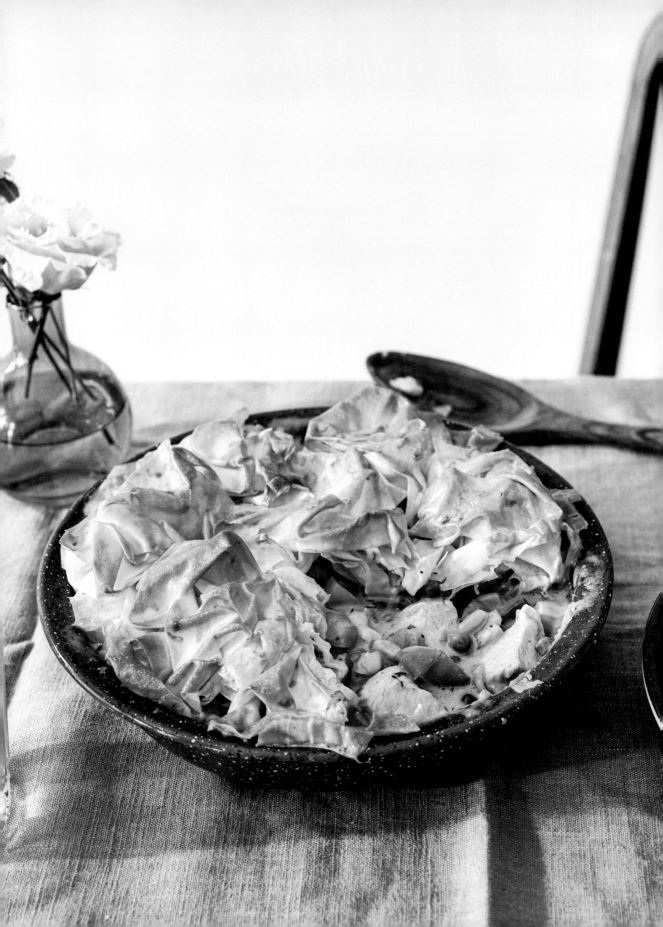

127
Calories

DF

Huli Huli Chicken with Spicy Grilled Pineapple

KCALS
127

FAT
4.5g

SAT FAT
1.2g

CARBS
8.6g

SUGARS
8.2g

FIBRE
0.8g

PROTEIN
12.7g

SALT
0.77g

MAKES 14 DRUMSTICKS
(NUTRITIONAL ANALYSIS IS PER DRUMSTICK)

For the chicken:
14 skinless chicken drumsticks

For the huli huli marinade:
4 tablespoons soy sauce
4 tablespoons passata
2 tablespoons tomato purée (paste)
2 tablespoons brown sugar
½ tablespoon Worcestershire sauce
1 teaspoon onion powder
3 garlic cloves, crushed
2 teaspoons grated fresh ginger
120ml (4fl oz) pineapple juice
2 spring onions (scallions), sliced

For the grilled pineapple:
1 fresh pineapple, sliced
¼ teaspoon cayenne pepper
cooking oil spray
sea salt

Gluten-free:
Use gluten-free soy sauce and Worcestershire sauce.

Swap:
You could also use bone-in skinless chicken thighs.

Tip:
If you prefer, you can remove the rind and core of the pineapple and slice into rings to grill.

Huli Huli chicken is a popular Hawaiian-style dish – huli meaning to reverse or turn, which is exactly what we do with these tender chicken drumsticks, which are cooked with a delicious marinade and paired with spicy grilled pineapple.

1. Mix together all the ingredients for the marinade.

2. Put the chicken into a ziplock bag and add the marinade, making sure all the pieces of chicken are coated. Refrigerate overnight (or for at least 4 hours).

3. Preheat the oven to 180°C/160°C fan/350°F/gas 4 and line a baking tray with parchment paper.

4. Remove the drumsticks from the bag, reserving the leftover marinade, and place on the lined baking tray. Bake in the oven for 20 minutes.

5. Put the marinade into a small saucepan and heat until it thickens.

6. Once the chicken has cooked for 20 minutes, remove from the oven, turn the drumsticks over, brush them with the marinade, then put back into the oven and cook for another 20 minutes.

7. Remove, turn again and give a final brush with the marinade, then turn the heat up to 220°C/200°C fan/425°F/gas 7 for the last 10–15 minutes. The chicken should be sticky and golden.

8. While the chicken is in the oven, grill (broil) the pineapple. Place the pineapple and cayenne in a bag and mix around to ensure it's all coated. Heat a griddle pan over a medium heat. Spray with cooking oil and grill each pineapple slice for about 2 minutes each side, until it is golden and you can see grill marks. Season with a pinch of salt.

9. When the chicken is ready, remove it from the oven, sprinkle with the sliced spring onions and serve with the grilled pineapple and your choice of sides.

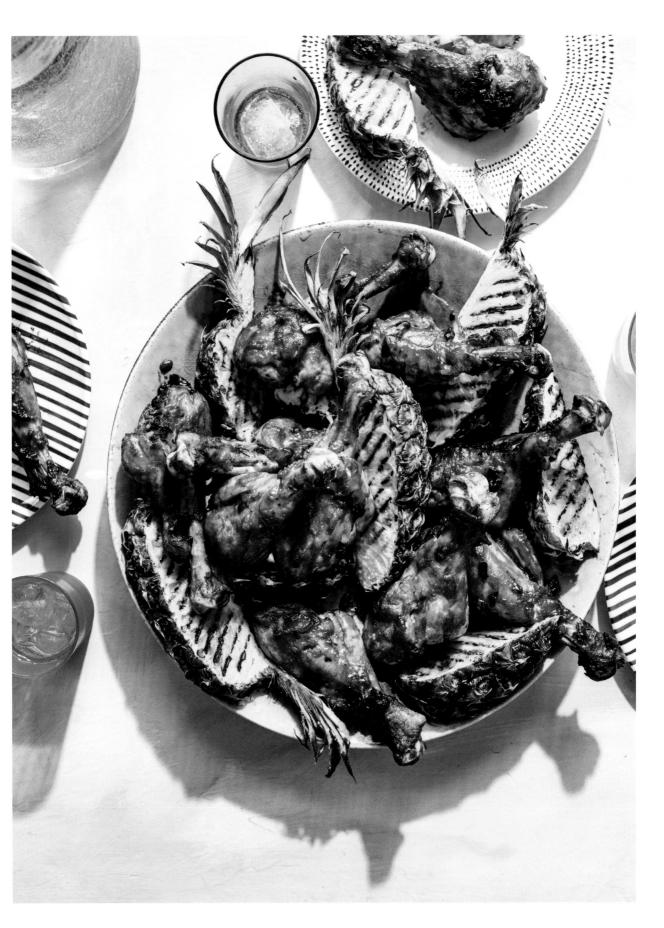

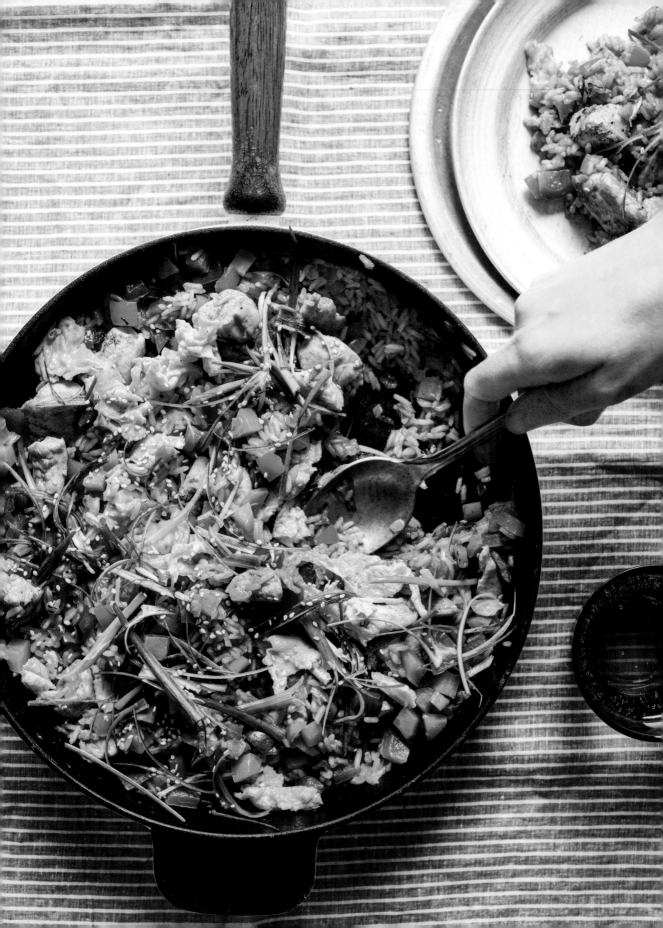

One-pot Firecracker Chicken Rice

SERVES 4

olive oil spray
300g (10½oz) skinless,
  boneless chicken (I use half
  breast, half thigh), diced
2 garlic cloves, crushed
salt and freshly ground
  black pepper
2 large eggs, beaten
1 onion, finely diced
1 small carrot, diced
1 red pepper, diced
1 green pepper, diced
2 tablespoons soy sauce
2 tablespoons sriracha
2 tablespoons brown sugar
2 tablespoons tomato purée
  (paste)
180g (6oz) long-grain rice,
  rinsed
480ml (17fl oz) chicken stock
2 spring onions (scallions),
  sliced
toasted sesame seeds
  (optional)

Gluten-free:
Use gluten-free soy sauce.

When I have had a busy day but I still want a tasty meal, fuss-free one-pot recipes like this firecracker chicken and rice with its sweet and spicy flavours are my saviour. I love the way all the ingredients are combined in one pot for minimum mess and clearing up.

1. Place a frying pan over a medium–high heat and spray with olive oil spray, then add the chicken and garlic, season with salt and freshly ground black pepper, and fry until golden. Remove from the pan and set aside.

2. Add the beaten egg and once it starts to set, break it up into pieces with a wooden spoon. Season with freshly ground black pepper and set aside.

3. Add the onion, carrot and peppers to the pan with more olive oil spray and fry until softened.

4. Return the chicken to the pan along with the soy, sriracha, brown sugar and tomato purée, and mix to coat.

5. Add the rice and stir until it is all coated.

6. Add the stock and bring to the boil, then reduce the heat, cover and simmer for approx. 12–15 minutes, until almost all the stock is gone (do not stir). Turn off the heat and leave untouched for 10–12 minutes.

7. Remove the lid and stir in the egg.

8. Sprinkle with sliced spring onions and sesame seeds, if using.

DF

KCALS
422

FAT
8.0g

SAT FAT
1.9g

CARBS
57.4g

SUGARS
19.5g

FIBRE
4.5g

PROTEIN
27.7g

SALT
2.48g

Butter Chicken Lasagne

KCALS
435

FAT
14.3g

SAT FAT
7.1g

CARBS
38.8g

SUGARS
10.9g

FIBRE
4.1g

PROTEIN
35.8g

SALT
0.90g

SERVES 6

For the chicken:
600g (1lb 5oz) skinless
    chicken breast
140g (5oz) plain fat-free
    yoghurt
2 teaspoons ground cumin
2 teaspoons ground coriander
1 teaspoon garam masala
1 teaspoon ground turmeric
1 teaspoon paprika
½ teaspoon Kashmiri
    chilli powder
1 tablespoon lemon juice
2 tablespoons butter

For the butter sauce:
cooking oil spray
160g (6oz) onions, diced
2 garlic cloves, crushed
2 teaspoons grated
    fresh ginger
½ teaspoon Kashmiri
    chilli powder
160g (6oz) butternut squash,
    peeled, then finely diced
    or grated
360ml (9½fl oz) chicken
    stock
250g (9oz) passata
1 red pepper, finely diced
salt and freshly ground
    black pepper

For the lasagne:
200g (7oz) dried oven-ready
    lasagne sheets (8 sheets)
300ml (10fl oz) 1% milk
1½ tablespoons cornflour
    (cornstarch)
15g (½oz) Parmesan, grated
salt and freshly ground
    black pepper
100g (3½oz) mozzarella,
    grated
chopped fresh coriander
    (cilantro)

Don't knock it until you try it. It may seem like a totally bizarre combination to turn butter chicken into a lasagne, but trust me – this really does work. It's an explosion of flavour.

1. Put the chicken, yoghurt, spices and lemon juice into a bowl, mix to combine, then refrigerate overnight (or for at least 4 hours).

2. To make the sauce, place a deep frying pan over a medium–high heat and spray with cooking oil. Add the onions and fry until softened, then add the garlic, ginger and chilli powder and fry for a further 30 seconds. Add the butternut squash and stock, bring to the boil, then cover and simmer until the butternut is soft (12–15 minutes).

3. Leave to cool a little, then transfer to a blender with the passata and blend until smooth.

4. Melt the butter in the frying pan over a medium–high heat, and add the chicken in a single layer, using tongs (if your pan is small, do this in 2 batches, using 1 tablespoon of the butter at a time).

5. As it starts to go golden underneath, flip it over and brown the other side of the chicken, being careful not to move it around the pan too much.

6. Once the chicken is all lightly golden, pour in the blended sauce, add the diced red pepper, and simmer for 5 minutes. Using a wooden spoon, break up the chicken breast into small pieces. Taste the sauce and add salt and freshly ground black pepper if needed.

7. Put half the chicken mixture into a 28 x 23cm (11 x 9 in) lasagne dish, top with 4 lasagne sheets, then add the rest of the chicken and top with the remaining 4 lasagne sheets.

8. Put the milk and cornflour into a small saucepan and gently heat, whisking, until it starts to thicken. Add the Parmesan and whisk until melted, then season with a little salt and freshly ground black pepper. Pour this sauce over the lasagne and sprinkle with the mozzarella.

9. Bake in the oven at 200°C/180°C fan/400°F/gas 6 for 30 minutes, by which time the top should be golden. Serve sprinkled with fresh coriander.

Freezing:
To reheat after freezing, warm through in an oven preheated to 180°C/160°C fan/350°F/gas 4.

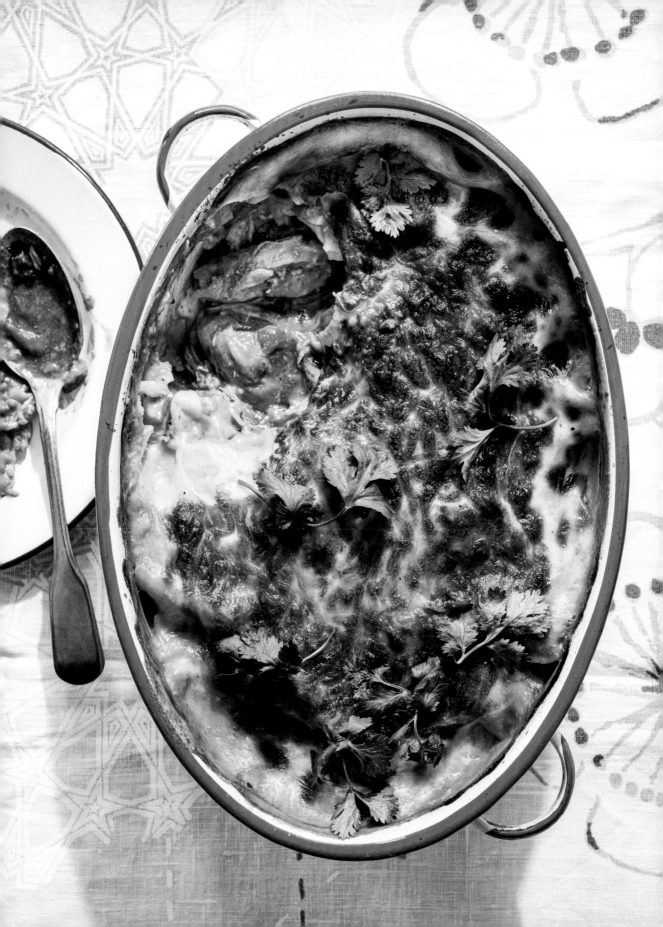

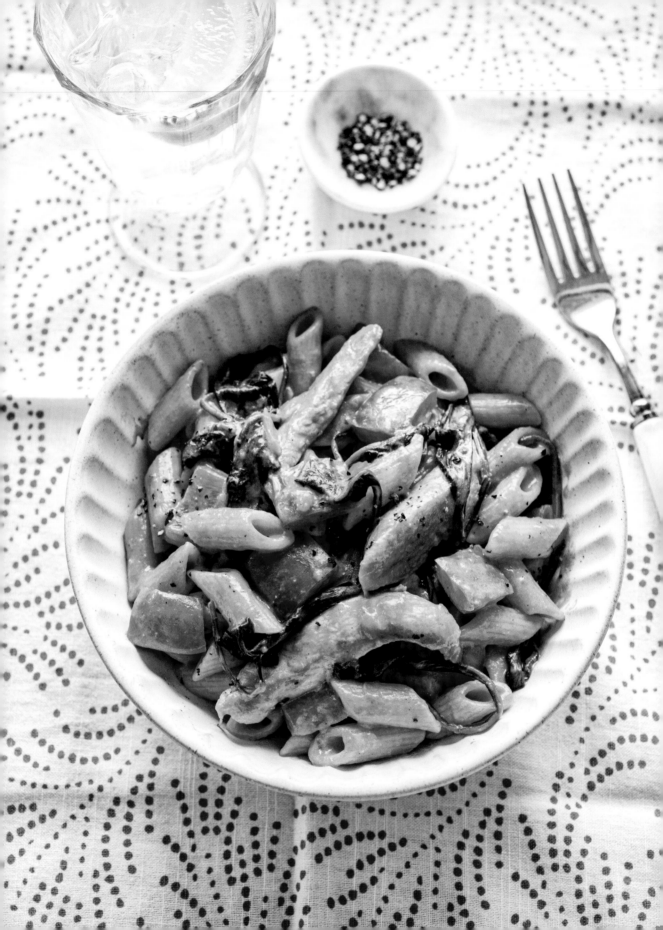

Creamy Red Pepper Penne with Chicken

SERVES 4

olive oil spray
400g (14oz) boneless
  skinless chicken breast,
  sliced
salt and freshly ground
  black pepper
1 tablespoon extra virgin
  olive oil
1 onion, diced
3 garlic cloves, crushed
2 large red peppers, diced
600ml (20fl oz) chicken
  stock
3 tablespoons tomato purée
  (paste)
240g (8½oz) dried
  penne pasta
60g (2oz) low-fat
  cream cheese
1 tablespoon chopped
  fresh basil
1 tablespoon chopped
  fresh parsley
15g (½oz) Parmesan, grated
4 handfuls of fresh spinach,
  stalks removed, roughly
  chopped

Serving side:

Pair with a simple mixed
salad.

Vegetarian:

You could swap out the
chicken for a vegetarian
chicken substitute (like soya
pieces or seitan) and use
vegetable stock instead of
chicken stock.

Sometimes it may seem daunting to make a homemade sauce for pasta, and it can be tempting to just open a jar. This creamy penne will be your go-to recipe for a simple pasta dish. Tender pieces of chicken in a yummy creamy red pepper sauce.

1. Place a frying pan over a medium–high heat and spray with olive oil. Add the chicken, season well with salt and freshly ground black pepper, and fry until golden. Remove from the pan and set aside.

2. Add the olive oil to the pan. Add the onion and fry until lightly golden, then add the garlic and peppers and fry for a further minute.

3. Slowly add 120ml (4fl oz) of the stock and cook to reduce down around the peppers and onion.

4. Add the tomato purée and stir to coat, then pour in the rest of the stock, bring to the boil and simmer for 10 minutes. Leave to cool a little, set some aside then place the rest in a blender and blend until smooth.

5. Cook the pasta in boiling salted water until al dente, then drain, reserving 60ml (2fl oz) of the pasta water.

6. Return the blended sauce to the frying pan and stir in the cream cheese, until it is all melted and combined.

7. Put the chicken back into the pan, along with the fresh basil and parsley. Then add the cooked pasta, the Parmesan and the reserved pasta water, and stir until the sauce is glossy and coats the pasta. Add the spinach and reserved peppers and stir until wilted.

8. Taste and season as required with salt and freshly ground black pepper. Divide between 4 bowls and enjoy!

KCALS
471

FAT
9.7g

SAT FAT
1.8g

CARBS
52.3g

SUGARS
8.9g

FIBRE
7.0g

PROTEIN
40.0g

SALT
1.17g

Umami Chicken Traybake

DF

KCALS
252

FAT
11.4g

SAT FAT
2.8g

CARBS
11.5g

SUGARS
9.9g

FIBRE
2.2g

PROTEIN
24.8g

SALT
1.79g

SERVES 4

8 boneless skinless chicken thighs
300g (10½oz) portobello mushrooms, gills removed, sliced
cooking oil spray (I used avocado)
2–3 spring onions (scallions), thinly sliced lengthways

For the umami paste:
2 tablespoons soy sauce
2 tablespoons tomato purée (paste)
½ tablespoon fish sauce
2 teaspoons paprika
2 garlic cloves, crushed
1 teaspoon sesame oil
1 tablespoon rice vinegar
1½ tablespoons maple syrup
white pepper

Low-carb side suggestions:
Special fried cauliflower rice (page 239), or sautéed shredded vegetables such as cabbage or beansprouts.

Gluten-free:
Use gluten-free soy sauce.

Side suggestion:
Serve with some cooked jasmine rice and additional stir-fried veggies of choice.

Umami means 'pleasant savoury taste', and when it comes to flavour this chicken dish with portobello mushrooms and spring onions ticks all the boxes. The fish sauce might seem like an odd ingredient, but trust me when I say the ingredient itself might smell fishy, but the flavour is anything but – it adds a deep, savoury umami explosion of taste to this traybake, especially when combined with all the other ingredients.

1. Preheat the oven to 200°C/ 220°C fan/425°F/gas 7 and line a large baking tray with parchment paper.

2. Mix the ingredients for the umami paste together, then put into a bowl with the chicken and toss to coat.

3. Place the chicken on the baking tray, evenly spaced out. Scatter the mushrooms in between.

3. Spray the chicken and mushrooms with cooking oil and bake for 35–40 minutes, taking the tray out halfway and brushing the chicken with all the juices.

4. Serve sprinkled with the spring onions and your choice of side.

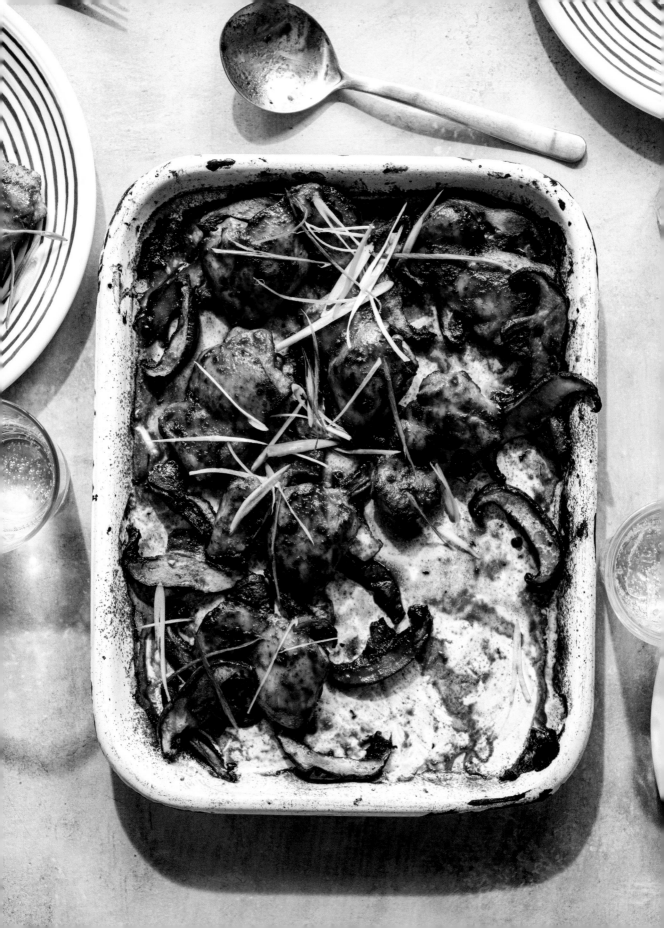

Chicken Greek Gyro Bowls

GF

KCALS
526

FAT
13.3g

SAT FAT
3.3g

CARBS
50.8g

SUGARS
12.3g

FIBRE
9.8g

PROTEIN
45.8g

SALT
2.53g

SERVES 4

600g (1lb 5oz) boneless
   skinless chicken thighs
1 medium onion, halved
   and sliced
olive oil spray
1 head of romaine lettuce,
   chopped
1 cucumber, sliced
24 cherry tomatoes, halved
1 small red onion, sliced
homemade hummus
   (see page 236)
1 lemon, quartered

For the seasoning:
2 tablespoons fat-free
   Greek yoghurt
1 tablespoon paprika
2 garlic cloves, crushed
2 teaspoons ground coriander
1 teaspoon ground cumin
1 teaspoon dried oregano
juice and zest of ½ a lemon
¼ teaspoon cayenne pepper
salt and freshly ground
   black pepper

For the tzatziki:
180g (6oz) fat-free Greek
   yoghurt
150g (5½oz) cucumber,
   grated (squeeze out
   excess liquid)
2 garlic cloves, crushed
1 tablespoon fresh dill
juice and zest of ½ lemon
1 teaspoon extra virgin olive
   oil, to drizzle on top

For the parsley rice:
180g (6oz) long-grain rice
480ml (17fl oz) chicken stock
2 tablespoons finely chopped
   fresh parsley

Enjoy a fakeaway night with these delectable chicken gyro bowls – tender seasoned oven-baked chicken with parsley rice, hummus, sautéed chickpeas, salad and tzatziki. Yes please!

1. Place the chicken, all the seasoning ingredients and 1 teaspoon salt and a pinch of freshly ground black pepper in a ziplock bag, toss to coat and place in the fridge overnight.

2. Preheat the oven to 220°C/ 200°C fan/425°F/gas 7 and line a baking tray with parchment paper.

3. Place the chicken thighs on the lined tray and scatter over the sliced onion. Spray the top with olive oil.

4. Bake for about 25 minutes, until golden and caramelized, then remove from the oven and slice (I like to place the slices under the grill (broiler) for a few minutes to char the edges, but this is optional).

5. Rinse the rice under running water in a colander until the water runs clear.

6. Place a saucepan over a medium–high heat and spray with olive oil. Add the rice and fry for about a minute, just until it goes translucent (watch it doesn't burn).

7. Pour in the stock, bring to the boil, then reduce the heat and simmer until the stock is almost gone (do not stir while cooking). Turn off the heat, put a lid on the pan and leave for 10–12 minutes.

8. Remove the lid and stir in the chopped parsley.

9. Mix the tzatziki ingredients, apart from the olive oil, together in a bowl (this can be prepared the day before). Drizzle over the extra virgin olive oil before serving.

10. Build your bowls: rice, chicken, lettuce, cucumber, tomatoes, red onion, homemade hummus and tzatziki. Serve with lemon quarters alongside. Delish!

Lower-carb side: Swap the rice for special fried cauliflower rice (page 239), or omit the rice and serve with extra salad.

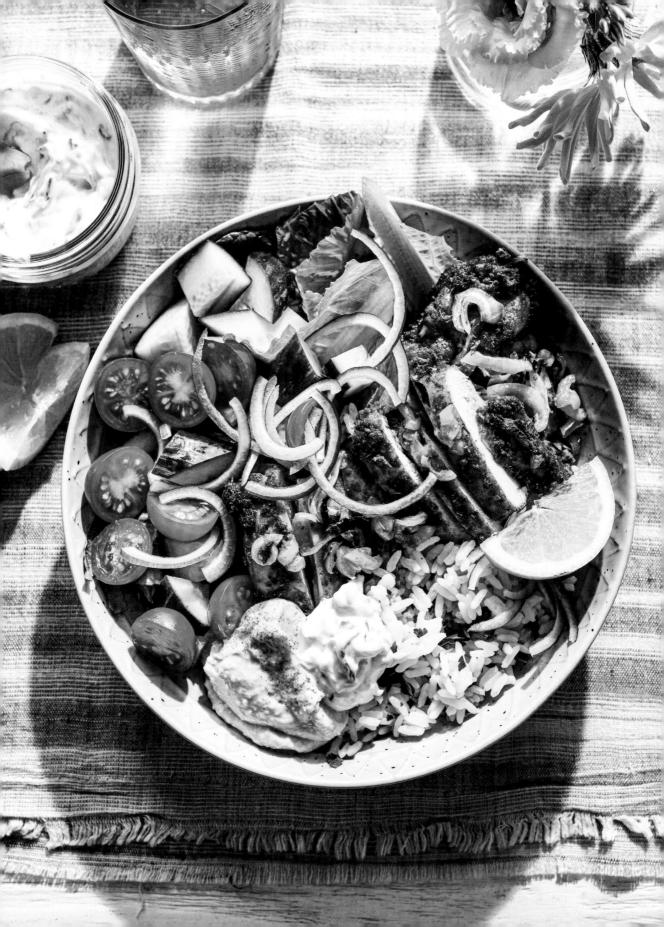

Chilli Lime Chicken and Rice Bake

KCALS
432

FAT
9.7g

SAT FAT
2.6g

CARBS
48.6g

SUGARS
6.0g

FIBRE
7.8g

PROTEIN
33.8g

SALT
1.93g

SERVES 4

8 bone-in skinless chicken
  thighs (all visible fat
  trimmed off)
2 tablespoons paprika
salt and freshly ground
  black pepper
1 teaspoon garlic powder
1 teaspoon onion powder
½ teaspoon ground coriander
½ teaspoon ground cumin
½ teaspoon cayenne pepper
juice of 1 small lime
180g (6oz) long-grain rice,
  rinsed
100g (3½oz) frozen
  sweetcorn
200g (14oz) tin of
  black beans
1 onion, halved and thinly
  sliced
3 garlic cloves, crushed
1 red pepper, diced
1 tablespoon tomato purée
  (paste)
420ml (14fl oz) chicken stock
olive oil spray
chopped fresh coriander
  (cilantro)
2 spring onions (scallions),
  sliced
lime wedges, to garnish

Some days I just want an easy meal I can throw into the oven, with minimum effort, and this is one of those recipes. Although it contains quite a few ingredients, once everything is all put together it is just a case of baking in the oven and it's done. As a family we love this served in the middle of the table with a bowl of soured cream, avocado and a simple salad, where we can just all dig in and help ourselves.

1. Preheat the oven to 200°C/180°C fan/400°F/gas 6.

2. Put the chicken into a bowl with the paprika, 1 teaspoon of salt, a pinch of freshly ground black pepper, the garlic powder, onion powder, coriander, cumin, cayenne and lime juice and mix to coat the chicken evenly.

3. Put the rice, sweetcorn, black beans, onion, garlic, red pepper and a little salt and freshly ground black pepper into a large baking dish.

4. Whisk the tomato purée into the stock and pour this over the rice, stirring to combine.

5. Place the chicken pieces on top, spray with olive oil spray then cover with foil, place in the oven and bake for 20 minutes.

6. Remove the foil and bake for a further 30 minutes.

7. Sprinkle with coriander and spring onions, and garnish with lime wedges.

Tip:
I don't recommend using boneless chicken or chicken breast for this recipe, as you will need to adjust the liquid. Using bone-in chicken ensures the correct ratio of stock/juices to cook the rice.

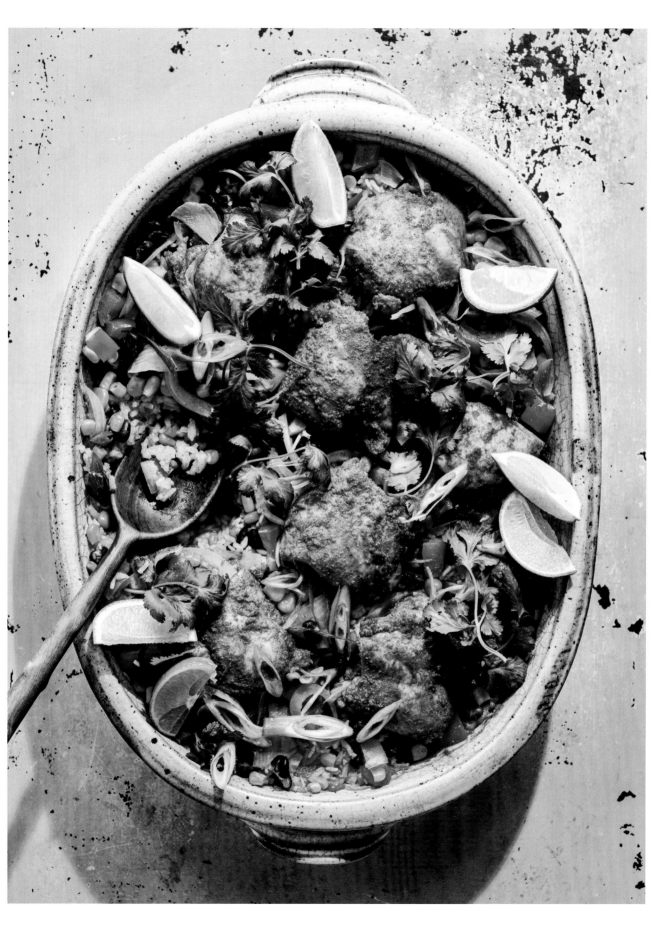

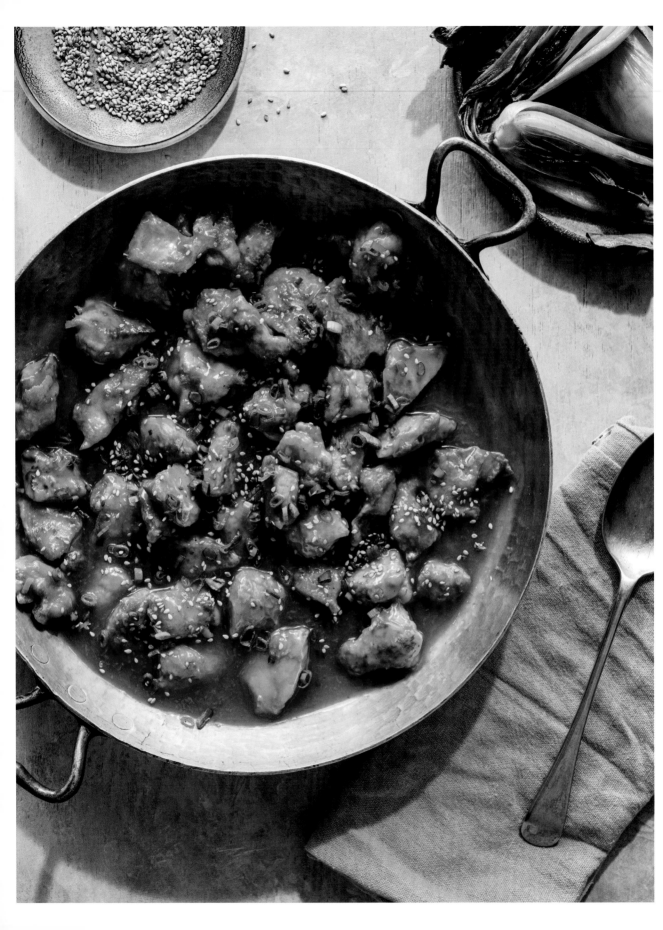

Orange Chicken

SERVES 4

600g (1lb 5oz) boneless
   skinless chicken thighs,
   sliced into bite-sized pieces
1 egg, beaten (but only
   use half)
3 tablespoons cornflour
   (cornstarch)
pinch of salt
cooking oil spray
2 spring onions (scallions),
   finely chopped
toasted sesame seeds

For the orange sauce:
180ml (6fl oz) orange juice
180ml (6fl oz) chicken stock
2 tablespoons soy sauce
4 tablespoons granulated
   sweetener
1 tablespoon cornflour
   (cornstarch)
zest of 1 orange
2 garlic cloves, crushed
½ tablespoon grated
   fresh ginger
pinch of red chilli flakes (add
   as much as you like to your
   desired spice level)

Gluten-free:
Use gluten-free soy sauce
and cornflour.

Swap:
If you prefer, you can swap
the sweetener for honey,
maple syrup or brown sugar.

Low-carb side suggestions:
Special-fried cauliflower rice
(page 239), or stir-fried bok
choy/cabbage or vegetables.

Orange chicken is one of my family's favourite take-out dishes, but that deep-fried coated chicken in sweet, sticky orange sauce can pack quite a few calories. This version is lightly coated and baked in the oven until golden before being stirred into a light orange sauce for a perfect fakeaway meal.

1. Preheat the oven to 230°C/ 210°C fan/ 450°F/gas 8 and line a baking tray with parchment paper.

2. Pat the chicken dry, then put it into a bowl with half the beaten egg. Toss to coat.

3. Add the cornflour and salt and mix until everything is combined and well coated.

4. Spread out on the lined tray, spray with cooking oil spray, and bake for 25–30 minutes, until crisp and golden, flipping the chicken over halfway through.

5. Put the orange sauce ingredients into a frying pan and simmer until they have thickened. Add the chicken and sprinkle with chopped spring onions and a pinch of sesame seeds.

DF

KCALS
279

FAT
9.8g

SAT FAT
3.0g

CARBS
20.5g

SUGARS
5.4g

FIBRE
0.6g

PROTEIN
27.0g

SALT
1.51g

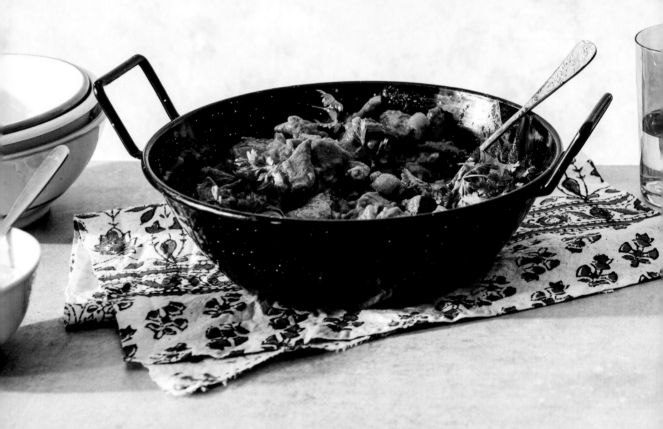

Meat

Thai Basil Pork

Cheeseburger
Meatzza

Steak Fajita Bowl

Thai Sweet Chilli
Pork Burgers

Philly Cheesesteak
Fries

Sesame Ginger Beef
with Noodles

Sloppy Joe Pie

Brunswick Stew

Mediterranean Beef
Meatballs with Olives

Ćevapi with Flatbreads
and Ajvar

Million Dollar Spaghetti

Slow Cooker Beef
and Apricot Tagine

Maple Balsamic Pork
Tenderloin with Roasted
Broccoli and Sweet Potato

BBQ Bacon Sweet
Potato Sliders

Lamb Balti Curry

219 Calories

Thai Basil Pork

SERVES 4

cooking oil spray
500g (1lb 2oz) extra lean
  (5% fat) pork mince
4 garlic cloves, crushed
1–2 red Thai chillies, sliced
1 red pepper, diced
3 spring onions (scallions),
  chopped
2 tablespoons soy sauce
  (reduced sodium
  if you prefer)
1 tablespoon fish sauce
1 tablespoon oyster sauce
2 tablespoons maple syrup
  or honey
120ml (4fl oz) chicken stock
handful of Thai basil

Gluten-free:
Use gluten-free soy sauce
and oyster sauce.

Swaps:
You can substitute pork
mince with chicken/turkey
mince, or chicken pieces –
the sauce consistency is best
with maple syrup/honey,
but swap for granulated
sweetener if you prefer.

Substitute for Thai basil:
If you can't get Thai basil
you can replace it with some
regular basil and a few fresh
mint leaves.

Side suggestions:
Serve with a fried egg and
white jasmine rice, or for
a lower-carb option some
cauliflower rice (page 239).

A quick and easy, fragrant stir-fry with minced pork, red chillies and Thai basil that is ready and on the table in less than 20 minutes. It's my go-to recipe for its simplicity and amazing taste.

1. Place a frying pan or wok over a medium–high heat and spray with cooking oil spray. Add the pork and garlic and fry until the pork just starts to go golden on the edges.

2. Add the chillies, red pepper and spring onions and fry for a further minute.

3. Add the soy sauce, fish sauce, oyster sauce, maple syrup and stock, and bubble until it reduces down into a sauce that just coats the meat.

4. Add the Thai basil and toss to combine.

5. Serve and enjoy!

KCALS
219

FAT
6.4g

SAT FAT
2.3g

CARBS
11.2g

SUGARS
8.9g

FIBRE
1.3g

PROTEIN
28.4g

SALT
2.97g

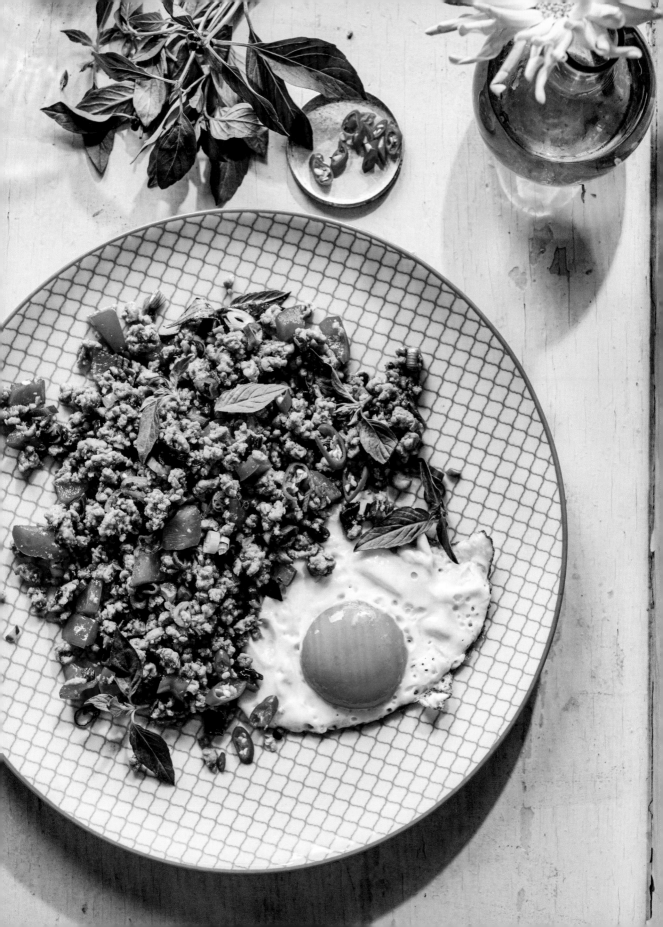

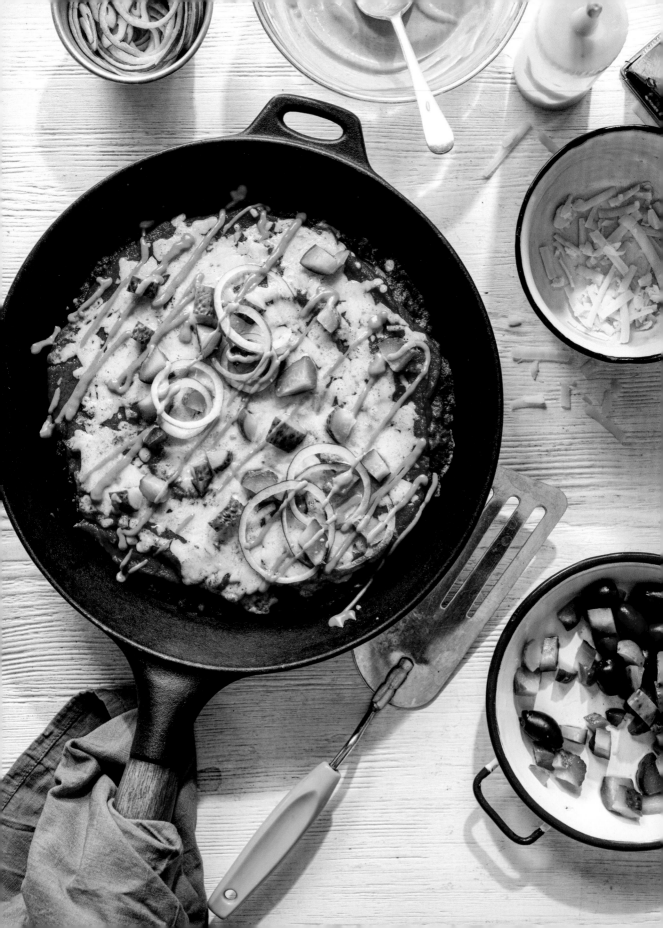

Cheeseburger Meatzza

SERVES 4

500g (1lb 2oz) extra
  lean (5% fat) beef mince
1 tablespoon cornflour
  (cornstarch)
salt and freshly
  ground black pepper
80g (3oz) passata
3 tablespoons tomato purée
  (paste)
1 teaspoon Worcestershire
  sauce
1 teaspoon paprika
½ teaspoon garlic powder
½ teaspoon onion powder
80g (3oz) Cheddar, grated
1 small onion, sliced
4 small gherkins, diced

For the burger sauce:
3 tablespoons light
  mayonnaise
1 tablespoon tomato purée
  (paste)
1 teaspoon yellow American
  mustard
pinch of garlic powder
pinch of onion powder
pinch of freshly ground
  black pepper
1 teaspoon granulated
  sweetener (optional)

Gluten-free:
Use gluten-free
Worcestershire sauce,
mustard and cornflour.

If you love anything cheeseburger-y, wait until you try my incredible cheeseburger meatzza. All the best components of a burger made into a meat-based pizza. Delicious, and a perfect recipe to enjoy with the whole family.

1. Preheat the oven to 220°C/ 200°C fan/425°F/gas 7.

2. Put the beef mince and cornflour into a bowl and mix until combined, then form into a large ball. Dust the outside of the ball with salt and freshly ground black pepper. Then put it into a round ovenproof dish (about 23–25cm/9–10 inches in width) and flatten it down.

3. Place in the oven and bake for 10 minutes, just until lightly browned.

4. Remove from the oven and dab up a little of the released juices if excessive (but not all – they keep the meat from drying out).

5. Mix together the passata, tomato purée, Worcestershire sauce, paprika, garlic powder and onion powder.

6. Spread this over the top of the patty, then top with the Cheddar.

7. Put back into the oven and bake for about 12–15 minutes, until the Cheddar is all melted and lightly golden.

8. Mix together all the ingredients for the burger sauce in a bowl.

9. Remove the patty from the oven and allow to rest for a few minutes.

10. Sprinkle the sliced onion and gherkins over the top, and drizzle over the burger sauce, then slice into 4 equal slices.

11. Serve with a mixed salad and enjoy.

GF

KCALS
587

FAT
22.1g

SAT FAT
9.0g

CARBS
50.3g

SUGARS
10.5g

FIBRE
9.8g

PROTEIN
41.8g

SALT
1.29g

Steak Fajita Bowl

SERVES 4

500g (1lb 2oz) flank steak
(or steak of your choice),
fat removed
salt and freshly ground
black pepper
olive oil spray
1½ green peppers, sliced into
strips
1½ red peppers, sliced into
strips
1 large onion, sliced into strips
75ml (2½fl oz) chicken stock

For the marinade:
2 garlic cloves
1 teaspoon ground cumin
1 teaspoon paprika
¼ teaspoon cayenne pepper
½ teaspoon sugar
1 tablespoon lime juice
½ teaspoon onion powder
1 jalapeño, deseeded
couple of tablespoons water
a small handful of coriander
(cilantro)

For the lime coriander rice:
180g (6oz) long-grain rice,
rinsed
450ml (16fl oz) chicken stock
2 tablespoons chopped fresh
coriander (cilantro)
juice and zest of ½ a lime

For the bowls:
romaine lettuce, chopped
4 tablespoons reduced fat
soured cream
120g (4oz) diced avocado
60g (2oz) Cheddar, grated

Who needs fajitas in tortillas when you can enjoy all the yummy components – lime coriander rice, peppers, soured cream, Cheddar and avocado – all in one bowl combo? Serve all the components in the middle of the table, so everyone can dig in, choose their favourite combo and celebrate the ultimate fajita night.

1. Put all the ingredients for the marinade into a mini food processor and do a couple of spins of the blade.

2. Put the steak into a shallow dish, season and cover with the marinade, ensuring it's rubbed all over, then refrigerate overnight.

3. When ready to cook, remove the steak from the dish and season the outside with salt. Spray a frying pan with olive oil and, once hot, add the steak and fry over a medium–high heat for 3 minutes per side (a little longer if you prefer your steak cooked more), then remove and set aside to rest.

4. Add the peppers and onion to the pan and fry for a couple of minutes, then gradually add the stock, reducing it down until all the stock is gone. Season with salt and freshly ground black pepper.

5. Put the rice and stock into a saucepan, bring to the boil, then cover the pan, reduce the heat and simmer until the stock is almost gone (do not stir). Turn off the heat and leave lidded for 10 minutes. The rice will be cooked perfectly. Stir in the coriander and the lime juice and zest.

6. Slice up the steak, then build your bowl: put some rice, steak, peppers, onion, romaine lettuce, sour cream, avocado and Cheddar into each bowl, or build your own combinations.

Low-carb suggestion:
Swap the lime coriander rice for
cauliflower rice (page 239) or
serve with a mixed salad.

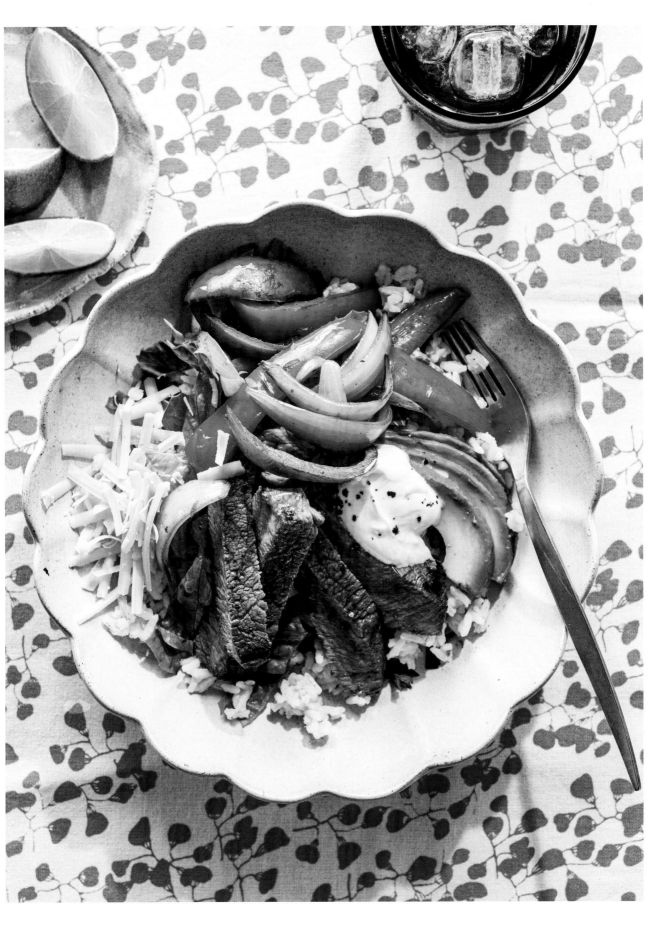

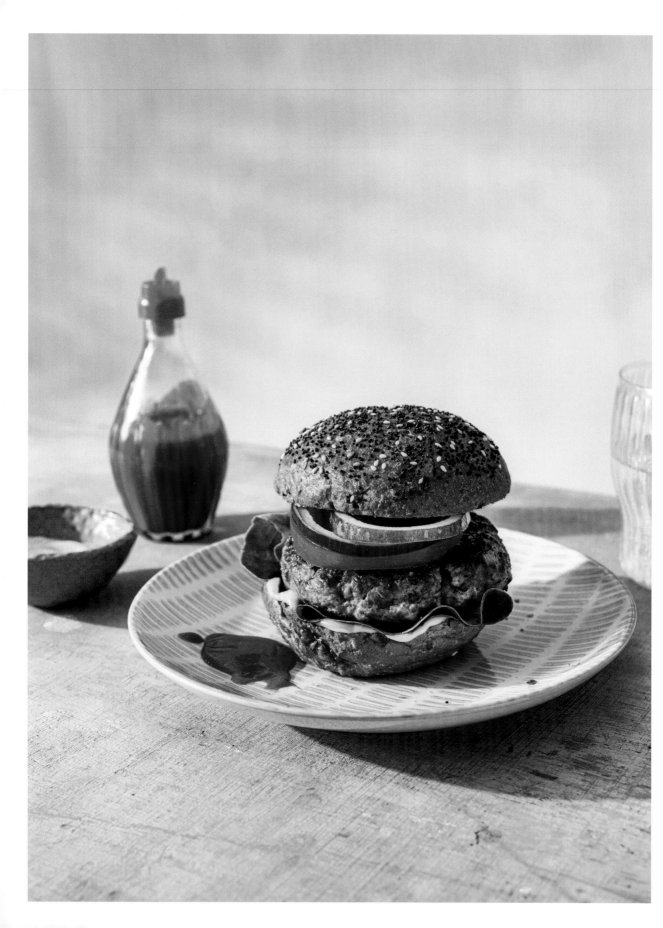

Thai Sweet Chilli Pork Burgers

SERVES 4

455g (1lb) extra-lean 5% fat
  pork mince
3 tablespoons Thai sweet
  chilli sauce
3 spring onions (scallions),
  chopped (green part only)
a handful of fresh coriander
  (cilantro), finely chopped
½ teaspoon garlic powder
½ teaspoon onion powder
pinch of red chilli flakes
  (optional for extra heat)
pinch of salt
cooking oil spray
4 small wholemeal (whole
  wheat) buns, lightly toasted
lettuce (I use butterhead/
  Boston lettuce)
tomato slices
red onion slices
low-fat mayo

Low-carb suggestion:
Serve these in lettuce wraps
with the toppings instead of
on bread rolls.

Gluten-free:
Use gluten-free bread rolls
and mayonnaise.

Swaps:
Minced chicken or turkey
also works well for this
recipe, but don't use any
less than 5% fat.

This burger recipe was one that came together by chance. So simple but totally delicious. With some minced pork to use up and nothing really planned for dinner, I just grabbed a few ingredients I had that I figured would go well together and what can I say... these yummy Thai sweet chilli pork burgers were born. A huge hit that I now make on regular rotation.

1. Combine the pork mince, sweet chilli sauce, spring onions, coriander, garlic powder, onion powder and a pinch of red chilli flakes in a bowl, then form into 4 equal-sized burgers. Season the outside of each burger with a little sea salt.

2. Spray a frying pan over a medium high heat with cooking oil spray, then add the burgers and fry for about 5–6 minutes each side, until golden and cooked through.

3. When the burgers are almost cooked, add the buns to the pan, cut side down, and just lightly toast.

4. Serve the burgers on the lightly toasted wholemeal buns, with lettuce and tomato slices, red onion slices and some low-fat mayo.

5. You can also make the mixture into 12 mini patties and enjoy them as a lighter meal with a salad.

Freezing:
Only the burger patties
are freezer-friendly. Freeze
after step 1. To reheat after
freezing, defrost in the fridge,
then follow steps 2–5. These
can also be frozen after
cooking.

KCALS
359

FAT
11.6g

SAT FAT
2.8g

CARBS
30.4g

SUGARS
9.4g

FIBRE
4.7g

PROTEIN
30.9g

SALT
1.19g

Philly Cheesesteak Fries

SERVES 4

800g (1lb 12oz) floury
    potatoes (I use russets)
cooking oil spray
2 teaspoons paprika
½ teaspoon garlic powder
salt and freshly ground
    black pepper
1 large onion, thinly sliced
1½ green peppers,
    thinly sliced
1 garlic clove, crushed
200g (7oz) mushrooms,
    sliced
240ml (9fl oz) beef stock
1 tablespoon Worcestershire
    sauce
350g (12½oz) sirloin steak
    (fat removed), thinly sliced
100g (3½oz) mozzarella,
    grated
2–3 gherkins, diced

Gluten-free:
Use a gluten-free
Worcestershire sauce.

The first time I ever had a Philly cheesesteak sandwich was all the way back in 2000, when I was working at a children's summer camp at the end of my three years at university. We went to a local diner and this leapt out at me on the menu. I regularly get cravings for it ever since. But all that steak, cheese and bread can be quite calorific. These Philly cheesesteak fries have all the taste but are much lighter on the calories.

1. Preheat the oven to 220°C/200°C fan/425°F/gas 7.

2. Slice the potatoes to your desired size of chips (fries) – I like to leave the skin on but you can peel them if you prefer.

3. Put the chips into a saucepan of water and bring to the boil. Once the water starts to bubble, turn off the heat, but leave the chips in the water for 3 minutes.

4. Drain the chips fully and blot dry with a clean kitchen towel.

5. Line a large baking tray with parchment paper and spray with cooking oil. Add the chips, paprika, garlic powder and ¾ teaspoon of salt, and toss to coat. Spread out evenly on the tray (to ensure even cooking), spray over the top with cooking oil spray, and bake for 40–45 minutes, until golden (flipping the chips over halfway through the cooking time). When they are close to being done, you can make the Philly cheesesteak.

6. Spray a frying pan with cooking oil, add the onion, peppers, garlic and mushrooms and fry for a couple of minutes to soften, then add a little of the stock at a time and reduce the vegetables until they are lovely and golden. Stir in the Worcestershire sauce.

7. Remove the vegetables from the pan and set aside.

8. Add the steak and a pinch of salt and freshly ground black pepper and stir-fry until cooked through. Return the vegetables to the pan and mix to combine.

9. Once the chips are cooked, remove from the oven and scatter the steak/veg mix on top. Add the mozzarella and sprinkle with the gherkins.

10. Place under the grill until the cheese is melted and lightly golden.

11. Dig in and enjoy!

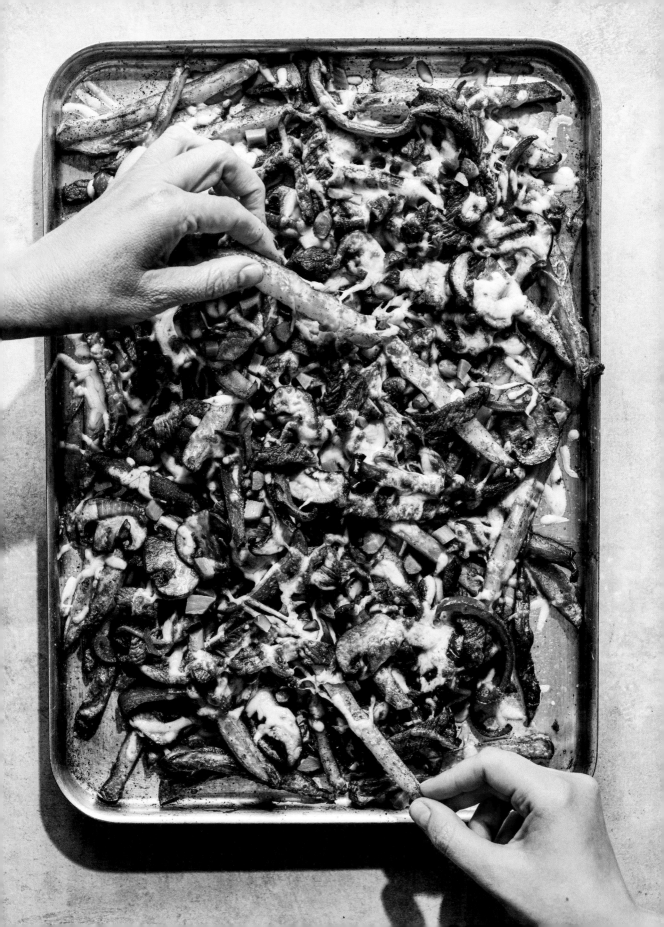

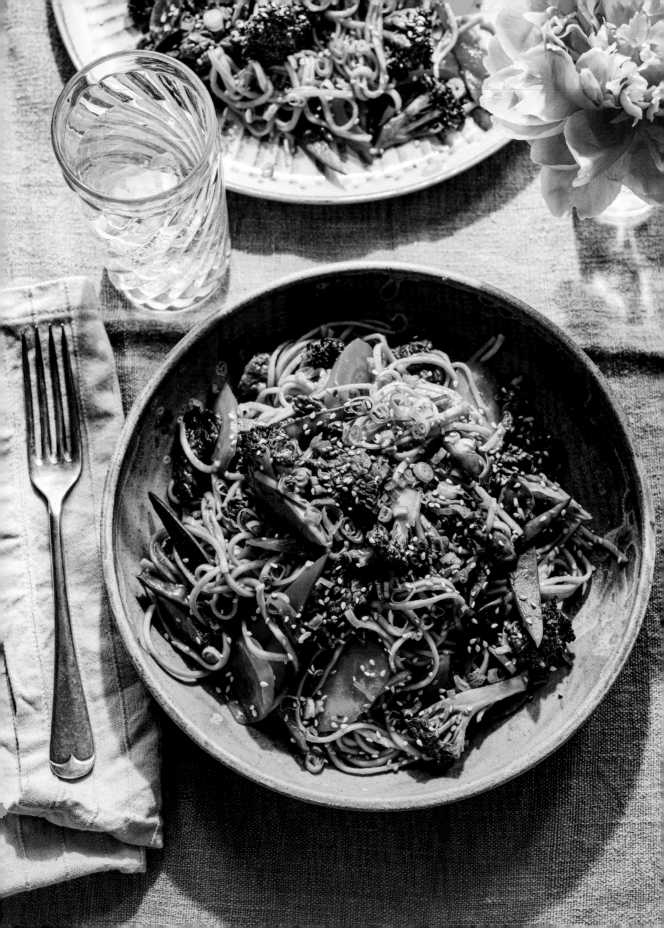

Sesame Ginger Beef with Noodles

404 Calories

SERVES 4

DF

400g (14oz) flank steak
(fat removed), thinly sliced
against the grain
2 garlic cloves, finely chopped
½ tablespoon grated
fresh ginger
cooking oil spray
175g (6oz) egg noodles
175g (6oz) broccoli,
broken into florets
175g (6oz) carrots,
cut into thin batons
1 red pepper, sliced
80g (3oz) mangetout
(snow peas)
1 tablespoon soy sauce
(reduced sodium)
2 tablespoons oyster sauce
1 tablespoon maple syrup
1 tablespoon rice vinegar
½ tablespoon sesame oil
4 spring onions (scallions),
sliced
1 teaspoon sesame seeds
pinch of freshly ground
black pepper

Create a comforting fakeaway at home with this flavoursome sesame ginger beef with noodles. Tender strips of steak and a rainbow of different vegetables and egg noodles, all finished off with the perfect sauce. A family favourite!

1. Fry the beef in a large frying pan or wok with the garlic and ginger with a spray of cooking oil until browned, then remove and set aside.

2. Cook the noodles according to the package instructions and drain. Set aside.

3. Fry the broccoli, carrots and red pepper in the frying pan with a little more oil spray for 2 minutes.

4. Add the mangetout, then add the beef and noodles and mix to combine.

5. Whisk together the soy sauce, oyster sauce, maple syrup, rice vinegar and sesame oil and add to the pan. Toss until all the ingredients are coated.

6. Sprinkle with chopped spring onions and sesame seeds, and a pinch of freshly ground black pepper if you like, then serve.

Gluten-free:
Swap the soy sauce, noodles and oyster sauce for gluten-free alternatives.

Vegetarian:
Swap out the beef for tofu and use a vegetarian oyster sauce substitute.

Swaps:
Don't fancy beef? Swap it for chicken (boneless thighs are best). This is great with a variety of different vegetables too, just keep the ratio around about the same.

KCALS
404

FAT
9.4g

SAT FAT
3.0g

CARBS
44.5g

SUGARS
9.4g

FIBRE
8.2g

PROTEIN
31.4g

SALT
1.62g

Sloppy Joe Pie

SERVES 6

400g (14oz) extra lean (5%) beef mince
1 onion, diced
2 garlic cloves, crushed
1 carrot, diced
1 red pepper, diced
1 green pepper, diced
180ml (6fl oz) beef stock
1 tablespoon tomato purée (paste)
180g (6oz) passata
1 tablespoon balsamic vinegar
½ tablespoon yellow American mustard
1 tablespoon paprika
1 tablespoon Worcestershire sauce
2 tablespoons brown sugar

For the potato topping:
600g (1lb 5oz) waxy potatoes
675ml (22fl oz) chicken stock
120g (4oz) Cheddar, grated
3 spring onions (scallions), sliced
60g (2oz) fat-free Greek yoghurt
salt and freshly ground black pepper
2 large eggs, beaten

Gluten-free:
Use gluten-free Worcestershire sauce and mustard.

Vegetarian:
Use a vegetarian mince alternative and vegetable stock.

Swap:
You can swap the sugar for granulated sweetener.

KCALS 360	
FAT 12.7g	
SAT FAT 6.5g	
CARBS 29.0g	
SUGARS 13.9g	
FIBRE 5.1g	
PROTEIN 29.9g	
SALT 1.49g	

Sloppy Joe (minced beef in a sweet, tangy tomato sauce) was another dish I first tasted when working at a children's summer camp in the US back in 2000, and I've been making my own healthier version ever since. It's now one of my kids' favourites, and is traditionally served in a bread (burger) bun, hence the 'sloppy' name (it can be messy to eat). Here I turn the sloppy Joe meat into a pie with inspiration from a traditional cottage pie and the result is excellent!!

1. Heat a frying pan over a medium–high heat. Add the beef mince, onion, garlic and carrot and fry until the mince is browned and the vegetables are softened.

2. Add the peppers, stock, tomato purée, passata, balsamic vinegar, mustard, paprika, Worcestershire sauce and sugar. Bring to the boil, then reduce the heat to medium, cover the pan, and simmer for 10 minutes. Set aside.

3. Preheat the oven to 200°C/180°C fan/400°F/gas mark 6.

4. Put the potatoes into a saucepan, cover with the stock, bring to the boil and simmer until soft.

5. Drain, then mash until smooth and then add two-thirds of the Cheddar, the spring onions and yoghurt and mix until combined. Season with salt and black pepper, then add the eggs and mix to combine.

6. Put the sloppy Joe mix into a 23cm (9 inch) round oven dish or other similar-sized dish.

7. Roughly spoon the mashed potatoes over the top, then add the rest of the grated Cheddar.

8. Bake in the oven for 30 minutes, until the cheese is melted and lightly golden.

9. Leave to rest for 10 minutes, then serve.

Freezing:
To reheat after freezing, defrost in the fridge then warm through in an oven preheated to 180°C/160°C fan/350°F/gas 4.

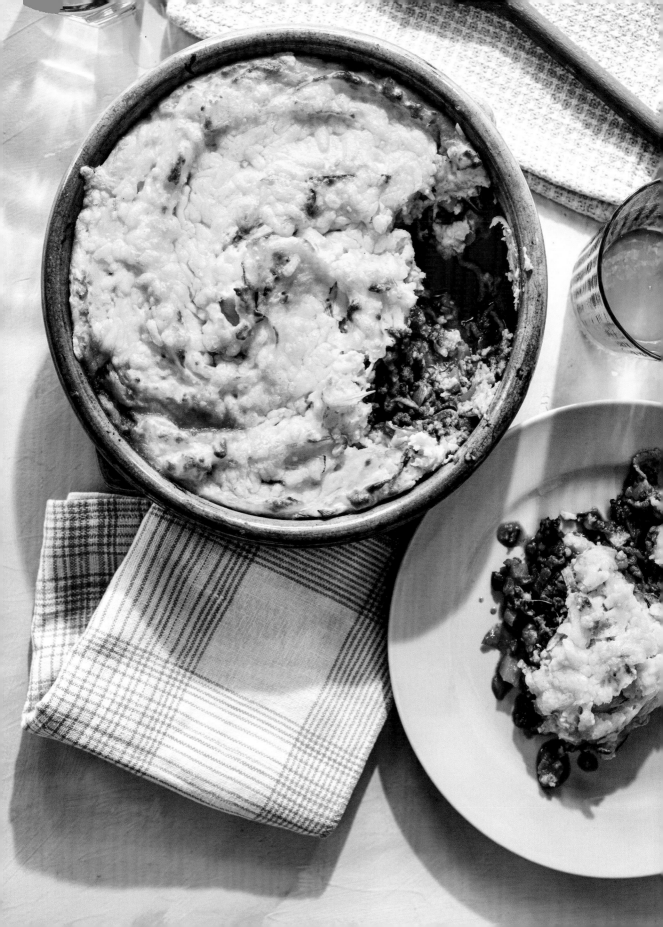

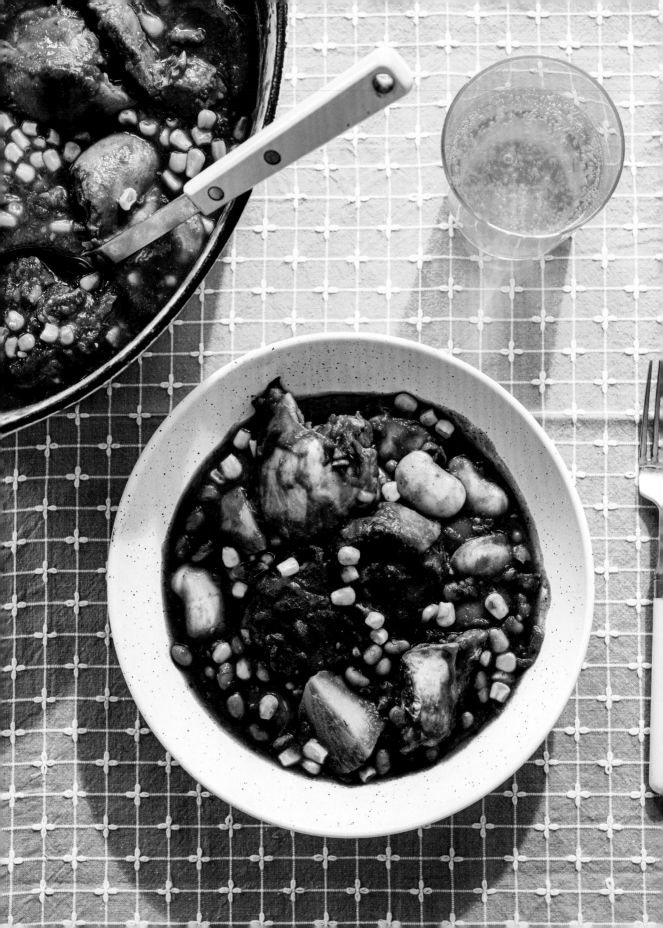

Brunswick Stew

SERVES 8

olive oil spray
700g (1lb 9oz) pork shoulder, fat removed
salt and freshly ground black pepper
1 large onion, sliced
3 garlic cloves, crushed
1½ tablespoons paprika
1 teaspoon smoked paprika
pinch of cayenne pepper, if you like it spicy (optional)
1 teaspoon garlic powder
1 teaspoon onion powder
1 tablespoon yellow American mustard
3 tablespoons maple syrup
3 tablespoons balsamic vinegar
1 tablespoon Worcestershire sauce
2 tablespoons tomato purée (paste)
1 x 400g (14oz) tin of chopped tomatoes
1 x 400g (14oz) tin of baked beans in barbecue sauce
480ml (17fl oz) chicken stock
300g (10½oz) boneless skinless chicken thighs
125g (4½oz) frozen sweetcorn
200g (7oz) waxy potatoes, diced
1 x 400g (14oz) tin of butter beans, drained and rinsed

One of the great things about living in Canada, with easy access to the US, is that I have been able to taste and try so many different foods and cuisines, and a lot of my inspiration comes from something I have tried in a restaurant or seen on a menu when travelling. This classic southern US dish combines a smoky tomato sauce with beans, potatoes and meat – usually pork – either on its own or in a combination such as the pork and chicken thighs I use in my version.

1. Heat a large casserole dish over a medium–high heat and spray with olive oil.

2. Season the outside of the pork shoulder with salt and freshly ground black pepper and fry until lightly golden. Set aside.

3. Spray the pan with a little more olive oil, then add the onion and fry until golden and softened. Add a little water to prevent burning if needed.

4. Add the garlic and fry for a further 30 seconds.

5. Add the spices, garlic powder, onion powder, mustard, maple syrup, balsamic vinegar, Worcestershire sauce and tomato purée and mix to combine.

6. Return the pork to the casserole with the tomatoes, baked beans and stock. Bring to the boil, cover, then reduce the heat and simmer for 2 hours.

7. Add the chicken thighs, frozen corn, potatoes and butter beans, and continue to simmer for an additional 45 minutes to 1 hour.

8. Taste and season as needed with salt and freshly ground black pepper.

9. Serve and enjoy with your choice of sides.

KCALS	**314**
FAT	**8.3g**
SAT FAT	**2.4g**
CARBS	**26.1g**
SUGARS	**13.0g**
FIBRE	**7.3g**
PROTEIN	**30.2g**
SALT	**0.97g**

Side suggestions:
Rustic kale and leek potato mash (page 255), or cauliflower cheese.

Lower-carb suggestion:
Mashed cauliflower, swede or celeriac (celery root).

Gluten-free:
Use gluten-free Worcestershire sauce and baked beans in barbecue sauce.

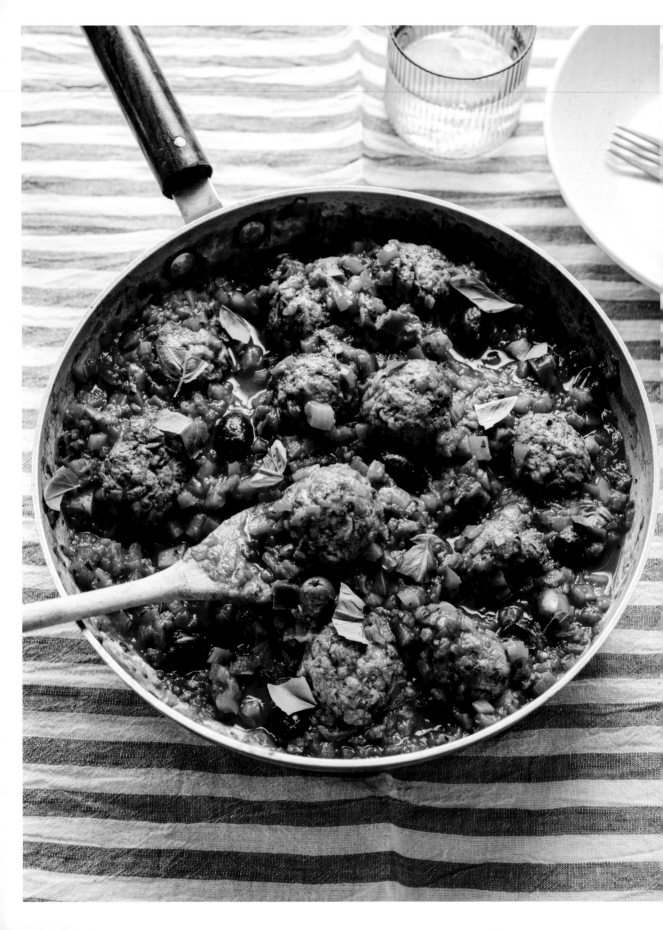

Mediterranean Beef Meatballs with Olives

285 Calories

SERVES 4

For the meatballs:
500g (1lb 2oz) extra lean (5% fat) beef mince
1 teaspoon garlic powder
1 courgette (zucchini), grated and excess liquid squeezed out
½ teaspoon onion powder
½ teaspoon garlic powder
1 tablespoon finely chopped fresh parsley
1 tablespoon tomato purée (paste)
1 teaspoon salt
pinch of freshly ground black pepper

For the sauce:
olive oil spray
1 onion, diced
3 garlic cloves, crushed
200g (7oz) aubergine (eggplant), chopped
125g (4½oz) carrot, chopped
1 red pepper, chopped
1 x 400g (14oz) tin of chopped tomatoes
2 tablespoons tomato purée (paste)
1 tablespoon balsamic vinegar
480ml (17fl oz) chicken stock
½ tablespoon granulated sweetener
1 teaspoon dried oregano
1 tablespoon chopped fresh basil
1 tablespoon chopped fresh parsley
½ tablespoon paprika
20 Kalamata olives, pitted
salt and freshly ground black pepper

It's funny how taste buds change the older you get. Olives are one of my addictions in adulthood – I hated them as a kid, but strangely I now can't get enough of them. So if I can add them to a dish, you'll be sure to see them featured, and they are a lovely addition to these flavoursome Mediterranean beef meatballs.

1. Preheat the oven to 180°C/160°C fan/ 350°F/gas 4 and line a baking tray with parchment paper.

2. Combine all the meatball ingredients together in a bowl. Form the mixture into 12 meatballs and put them on the lined tray. Bake for 10 minutes, then set aside.

3. Place a deep frying pan over a medium–high heat and spray with olive oil.

4. Fry the onion for a few minutes until translucent, then add the garlic, aubergine, carrot and red pepper and fry for a further couple of minutes until softened.

5. Add the tinned tomatoes, tomato purée, balsamic vinegar, stock, sweetener, herbs and paprika and bring to the boil, then reduce the heat, cover the pan and simmer for 25 minutes.

6. Add the meatballs and olives to the pan of sauce and simmer for an additional 15–20 minutes.

7. Season with salt and freshly ground black pepper.

8. Serve with your choice of sides. It's perfect over rice, pasta or mashed potatoes.

Lower-carb side suggestions:
Mashed cauliflower, courgette noodles or cauliflower rice.

Freezing:
Freeze the meatballs and sauce separately. To reheat, defrost in the fridge then warm through in a saucepan over a medium heat.

GF

DF

KCALS
285

FAT
8.0g

SAT FAT
3.1g

CARBS
15.4g

SUGARS
13.4g

FIBRE
7.5g

PROTEIN
34.3g

SALT
2.74g

Ćevapi with Flatbreads and Ajvar

SERVES 4

For the ćevapi:
300g (10½oz) extra lean (5% fat) beef mince
300g (10½oz) extra lean (5% fat) pork mince
¾ teaspoon bicarbonate of soda (baking soda)
1 teaspoon salt
½ teaspoon freshly ground black pepper
½ teaspoon red chilli flakes
1½ teaspoons paprika
2 tablespoons water
1 garlic clove, crushed

For the ajvar:
2 red peppers, sliced in half
250g (9oz) aubergine (eggplant), diced
1 garlic clove, crushed
2 teaspoons extra virgin olive oil
1 teaspoon white wine vinegar
pinch of salt and freshly ground black pepper

For the flatbread:
120g (4oz) plain (all purpose) flour
150g (5½oz) fat-free Greek yoghurt
½ teaspoon baking powder
pinch of salt
cooking oil spray

To serve:
red onion, sliced
fresh ripe tomatoes, sliced
garlic sauce (page 234)

Gluten-free:
Use a gluten-free bread.

Lower-carb suggestion:
Omit the flatbreads and serve with a salad.

KCALS	**417**
FAT	**11.6g**
SAT FAT	**3.6g**
CARBS	**31.7g**
SUGARS	**7.7g**
FIBRE	**5.4g**
PROTEIN	**43.9g**
SALT	**2.36g**

This was inspired by a local deli that sells the best homemade ćevapi with lepinja bread, ajvar sauce and garlic sauce with salad. I was introduced to this amazing food by a friend, and created my own lower-calorie version at home. It's a recipe you can serve at the table for everyone to help themselves.

1. Preheat the oven to 230°C/210°C fan/450°F/gas 8.

2. Combine the beef, pork, and the rest of the ćevapi ingredients in a bowl – don't over-mix.

3. Form into 16 equal-sized mini sausage shapes and place them on a plate. Cover them with clingfilm until ready to cook.

4. Place the peppers and aubergine on a baking sheet, cut side down, and roast for 25–30 minutes, until nice and charred. Remove from the oven, put into a bowl and cover tightly with clingfilm until the skin softens enough to peel off the peppers. Discard any large seeds from the aubergine and scoop out the flesh. Put the peppers and aubergine into a food processor with the garlic, oil, vinegar and some salt and pepper and pulse to a purée, adding a little water if needed. This can be served hot or cold.

5. For the flatbread, put the flour (reserve a little for dusting), yoghurt, baking powder and salt into a bowl. Combine with a silicone spatula or wooden spoon at first, until it all comes together, then knead with your hands until the side of the bowl is clear. Divide into 4 equal-sized balls. Take one ball, dust with a little flour and flatten between sheets of parchment paper. Roll into a flatbread, rotating and flipping with each roll, then place on a plate and repeat with the remaining 3 balls of dough.

6. Heat a pan over a medium–high heat. Spray with cooking oil and cook the flatbreads for about 3 minutes per side (they should be lightly brown in areas). Set aside.

7. Heat a griddle pan or a cast iron frying pan over a medium heat and spray with cooking oil. Add the ćevapi and cook until browned all over and cooked through, rotating them so they cook evenly. They will take about 12–15 minutes.

9. Take a flatbread, spread it with ajvar, top with the cooked ćevapi, red onion and tomatoes, and drizzle with the garlic sauce. Enjoy!

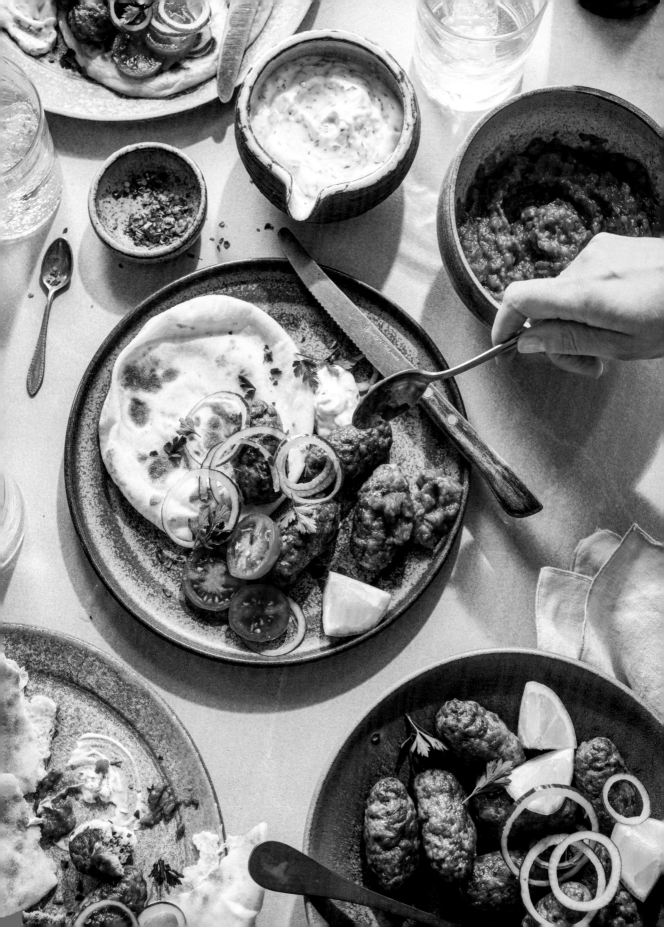

Million Dollar Spaghetti

SERVES 4

300g (10½oz) extra lean
(5% fat) beef mince
80g (3oz) onion, diced
1 garlic clove, crushed
180g (6oz) dried spaghetti
150g (5½oz) fat-free
cottage cheese
80g (3oz) light cream cheese
100g (3½oz) mozzarella,
grated

For the marinara sauce:
olive oil spray
80g (3oz) onion, chopped
80g (3oz) carrot, chopped
4 garlic cloves, crushed
1 x 400g (14oz) tin of
chopped tomatoes
1 tablespoon tomato purée
(paste)
240ml (9fl oz) chicken stock
a few torn fresh basil leaves
1 teaspoon dried oregano
salt and freshly ground
black pepper

Gluten-free:
Use gluten-free pasta.

Vegetarian:
Replace the beef mince with
a vegetarian mince and use
vegetable stock.

Side suggestions:
I pair this with a simple
salad (shredded romaine or
iceberg lettuce, cucumber,
red onion and tomatoes).

Swap:
You can replace the cottage
cheese with ricotta or
additional cream cheese.

KCALS	**434**
FAT	**10.6g**
SAT FAT	**5.9g**
CARBS	**45.1g**
SUGARS	**11.0g**
FIBRE	**5.1g**
PROTEIN	**37.0g**
SALT	**1.31g**

**I can only assume this dish gets its name because it literally
feels like a million dollars when you eat it – decadent, creamy,
cheesy and delicious. My kids come scrambling for seconds
whenever I make this. So if you are serving for 4, you may
want to double up the recipe for the ones who can't stop at
one serving. Traditionally it is quite a calorific dish, but with
a few healthy swaps this can be enjoyed by anyone who is
trying to eat a little more healthily or reduce their calories.**

1. Preheat the oven to 200°C/180°C fan/400°F/gas 6.

2. To make the marinara sauce, place a frying pan over a medium–
high heat and spray with olive oil. Add the onion, carrot and garlic
and cook until slightly softened.

3. Add the chopped tomatoes, tomato purée, stock and herbs,
bring to the boil, then cover the pan, reduce the heat and simmer
for 15 minutes. Allow to cool a little, then roughly blend. Season
with salt and freshly ground black pepper, and set aside.

4. Add the beef mince to the frying pan with the onion and garlic
and fry until browned.

5. Stir in half the marinara sauce and set aside.

6. Cook the spaghetti until al dente, drain, then put back into
the pan and stir in the other half of the marinara sauce.

7. Mix together the cottage cheese and cream cheese.

8. Place half the spaghetti in an ovenproof dish, then add the cottage
cheese mix and spread over the top with a spatula. Add the other
half of the spaghetti, top with the meat mixture, and sprinkle over
the mozzarella.

9. Bake in the oven for 30–35 minutes, until the cheese on top is
melted and golden.

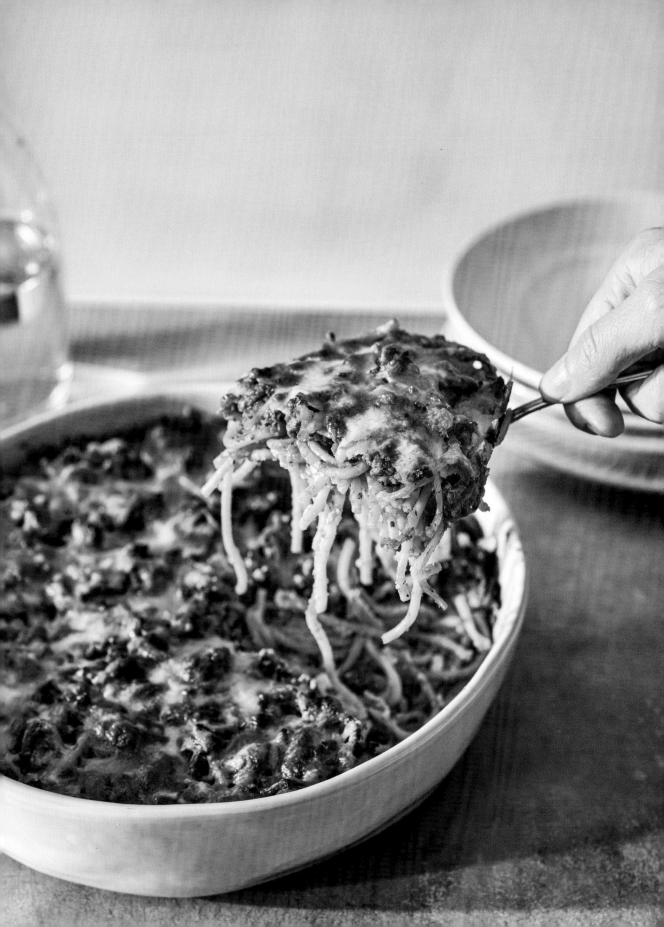

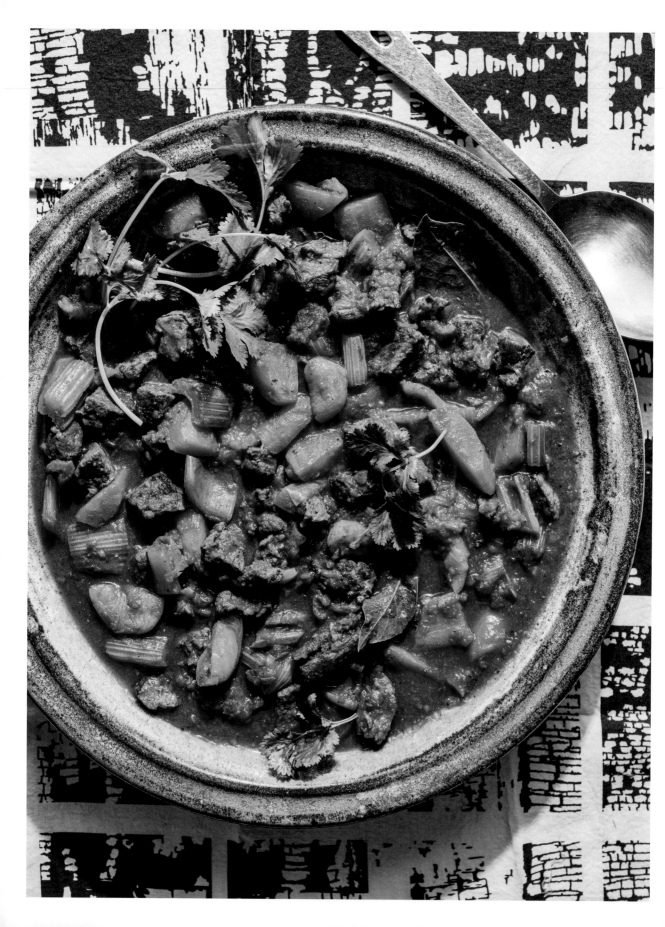

Slow Cooker Beef and Apricot Tagine

SERVES 4

olive oil spray
650g (1lb 7oz) diced lean
  beef (fat removed), diced
1 large onion, chopped
200g (7oz) celery, chopped
200g (7oz) carrots, diced
salt and freshly ground
  black pepper
5 garlic cloves, crushed
1 tablespoon paprika
2 teaspoons ground cumin
¾ teaspoon turmeric
1 stick of cinnamon (or
  ½ teaspoon ground
  cinnamon)
pinch of cayenne pepper, for
  some heat (optional)
a couple of bay leaves
75g (3oz) dried apricots
1 x 400g (14oz) tin of
  chopped tomatoes
2 tablespoons tomato purée
  (paste)
180ml (6fl oz) beef stock

To serve:
2 tablespoons chopped
  fresh coriander (cilantro)

Swaps:
Add 2½ tablespoons of
ras-el-hanout seasoning
instead of the spices. This
also works with diced lamb.

Side suggestions:
Couscous, cauliflower rice
(page 239) or mash.

Freezing:
To reheat after freezing,
simply defrost in the fridge,
then warm through in the
microwave or in a saucepan
over a medium heat.

Tender, slow-cooked chunks of beef with sweet apricots in an aromatic sauce with Moroccan-inspired spices. This is pure comfort in a bowl.

1. Heat a frying pan and spray with olive oil. Add the beef and brown it all over, then put into the slow cooker.

2. Spray the frying pan with a little more olive oil. Add the onion, celery and carrots and fry for a few minutes to soften.

3. Add a pinch of salt and the garlic and fry for a further minute or so.

4. Add to the slow cooker with the rest of the ingredients and mix to combine.

5. Set to slow-cook on low for 8 hours.

6. Once the tagine has finished cooking, taste and season with salt and black pepper. Before serving, stir in 2 tablespoons of chopped fresh coriander.

KCALS
365

FAT
11.3g

SAT FAT
4.2g

CARBS
22.7g

SUGARS
20.3g

FIBRE
8.8g

PROTEIN
38.8g

SALT
0.37g

BBQ Bacon Sweet Potato Sliders

KCALS
364

FAT
13.2g

SAT FAT
6.5g

CARBS
32.3g

SUGARS
18.6g

FIBRE
5.2g

PROTEIN
26.4g

SALT
1.26g

SERVES 4

300g (10½oz) extra lean (5% fat) beef mince
100g (3½oz) lean smoked bacon (fat removed), finely diced
1–2 large sweet potatoes, cut into 1cm (½ inch) slices (I leave the skin on) – you will need 8 slices in total
olive oil spray
1 teaspoon paprika
½ teaspoon garlic powder
½ teaspoon onion powder
salt and freshly ground black pepper
lettuce
4 Cheddar slices
sliced tomatoes
red onion slices
pickles

For the BBQ sauce
60g (2oz) passata
½ tablespoon tomato purée (paste)
2 tablespoons water
1 teaspoon Worcestershire sauce
1 teaspoon yellow American mustard
1 tablespoon balsamic vinegar
1 tablespoon maple syrup
½ teaspoon paprika
¼ teaspoon onion powder
¼ teaspoon garlic powder
¼ teaspoon smoked paprika

You won't miss the bun with these yummy BBQ bacon sweet potato sliders – the burgers are combined with pieces of smoky bacon and topped with a simple BBQ glaze, sandwiched between two baked seasoned sweet potato slices and your usual favourite toppings, such as Cheddar, lettuce and pickles.

1. Preheat the oven to 220°C/200°C fan/425°F/gas 7.

2. Combine the mince and chopped bacon in a bowl. Form into 4 burgers, then set aside.

3. Spray the sweet potato slices with olive oil, add the paprika, garlic powder and onion powder and toss to coat.

4. Place the sweet potato slices on a baking tray and bake for 30 minutes, until lightly golden (do not let them get too soft).

5. Put the BBQ sauce ingredients into a small saucepan and heat until the sauce thickens. Set aside.

6. Place a frying pan over a medium–high heat and spray with olive oil. Season the outside of the burgers with salt and freshly ground black pepper.

7. Cook the burgers until golden on both sides and cooked through.

8. Brush the tops of the burgers with the sauce until coated.

9. Build your sliders: place half the sweet potato slices on a plate. Add some lettuce, then a burger, then the cheese, and top with tomatoes, red onion slices and pickles.

Dairy-free:
Omit the cheese.

Gluten-free:
Use gluten-free Worcestershire sauce.

Serving suggestion:
These burgers can also be served in wholemeal (whole wheat) burger buns or with a mixed salad instead of sweet potato slices.

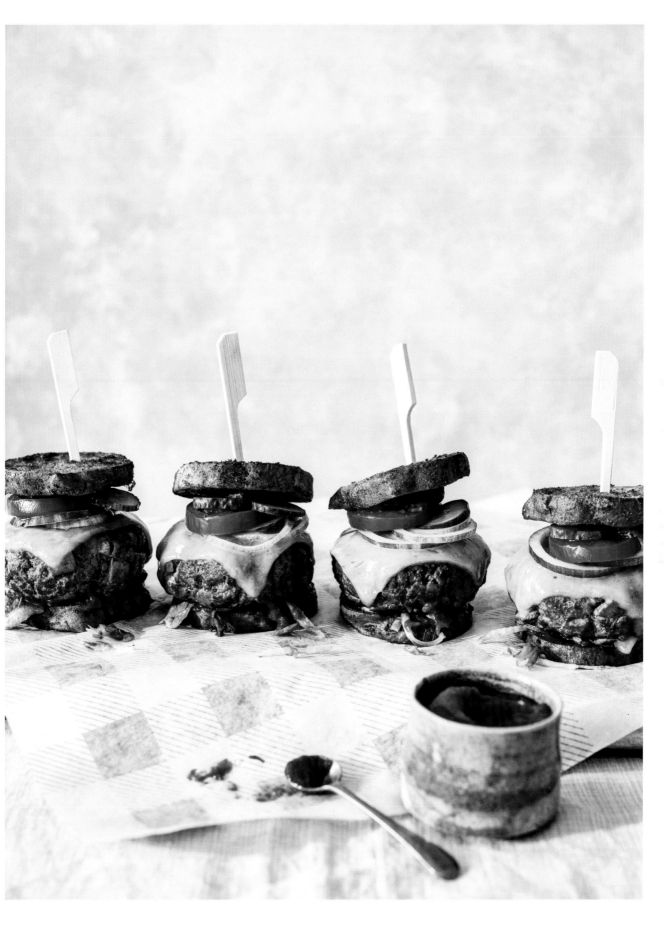

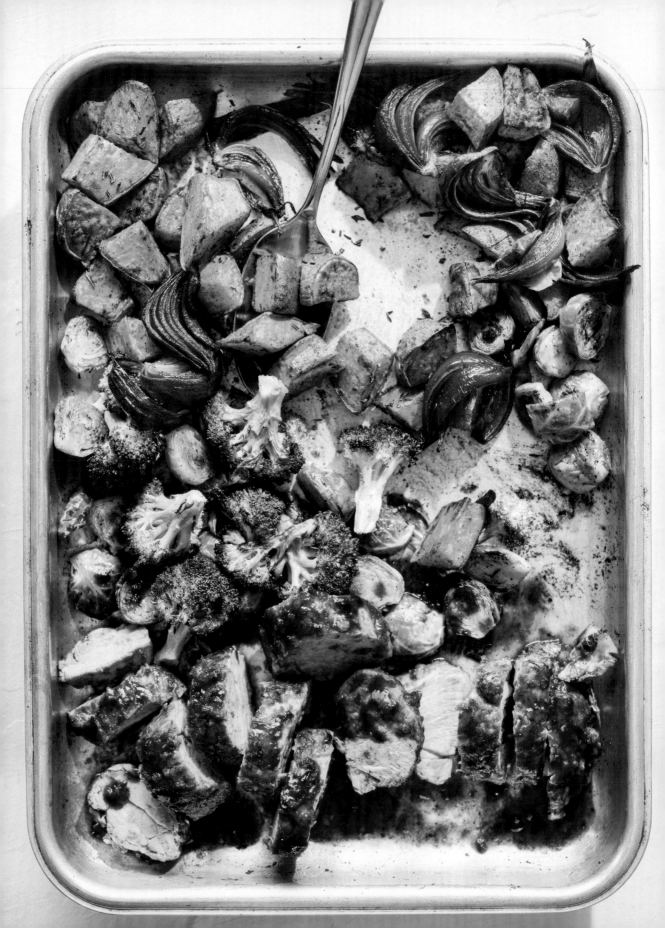

Maple Balsamic Pork Tenderloin with Roasted Broccoli and Sweet Potato

433 Calories

DF

SERVES 4

455g (1lb) sweet potato, cubed
1 red onion, halved and sliced
½ tablespoon paprika
1 tablespoon olive oil
650g (1lb 7oz) pork tenderloin (fillet), fat removed
1 tablespoon cornflour (cornstarch)
salt and freshly ground black pepper
cooking oil spray
4 tablespoons balsamic vinegar
2 tablespoons maple syrup
1 teaspoon garlic powder
120ml (4fl oz) chicken stock
455g (1lb) broccoli florets, brussels sprouts or mix of both
3 garlic cloves, crushed
½ tablespoon fresh thyme leaves, chopped
½ tablespoon fresh rosemary leaves, chopped

Gluten-free:
Use gluten-free cornflour.

Lower-carb suggestion:
Swap the sweet potatoes for cubes of butternut squash.

One of the great things about pork tenderloin is that it really doesn't take that long to cook, so with a few simple sides like roasted broccoli and sweet potato, you can have a quick and easy meal ready with minimum effort. Living in Canada, one of my favourite store cupboard ingredients is maple syrup, and with a little bit of balsamic vinegar it makes a stunning glaze that is ideal for this dish.

1. Preheat the oven to 220°C/200°C fan/425°F/gas 7.

2. Toss the sweet potatoes and onion with the paprika. Put on a baking tray with half the olive oil and bake for 25 minutes.

3. Dust the pork with the cornflour and season both sides with a pinch of salt and freshly ground black pepper. Spray a frying pan with cooking oil and place over a medium–high heat. Sear the meat until lightly golden, then remove and set aside.

4. Add the balsamic vinegar, maple syrup, garlic powder and stock to the pan in which you seared the pork, and heat until it becomes glaze-like (don't overheat or it will burn). Put the pork back into the pan and roll it around to fully coat. Place the pork and glaze on a piece of foil and roll the foil up around the pork to make a boat shape.

5. After 25 minutes move the sweet potatoes and onion over so they take up one third of the tray.

6. Put the broccoli in the middle of the tray with the crushed garlic, then drizzle the rest of the olive oil over the broccoli with a pinch of salt and black pepper and toss to coat.

7. Sprinkle the sweet potatoes and broccoli with the fresh thyme and rosemary.

8. Add the pork in its foil boat to the remaining third of the tray and put back into the oven for 20 minutes, until the pork is cooked through and the broccoli is cooked.

9. Let the pork rest for 10 minutes before slicing.

10. Serve the pork with the vegetables and drizzle with the glaze.

KCALS
433

FAT
8.8g

SAT FAT
2.2g

CARBS
44.6g

SUGARS
20.2g

FIBRE
12.6g

PROTEIN
37.5g

SALT
0.49g

Lamb Balti Curry

KCALS
321

FAT
16.9g

SAT FAT
6.7g

CARBS
12.1g

SUGARS
9.9g

FIBRE
4.9g

PROTEIN
30.0g

SALT
1.51g

SERVES 4

550g (1lb 4oz) diced lamb, trimmed of any visible fat.
50g (2oz) plain fat-free yoghurt
cooking oil spray
1 large onion, chopped
4 garlic cloves, crushed
1 tablespoon grated fresh ginger
salt and freshly ground black pepper
2 ripe tomatoes, chopped
½ teaspoon turmeric
1 teaspoon ground coriander
½ teaspoon garam masala
4 cardamom pods
1½ teaspoons Kashmiri chilli powder
1 green chilli, sliced in half lengthways
1 green pepper, sliced
1 red pepper, sliced
120g (4oz) passata
120ml (4fl oz) water
2 tablespoons chopped fresh coriander (cilantro)
½ tablespoon granulated sweetener (optional)

Lower-carb side:
Serve with cauliflower rice (page 239).

Gluten free:
Use gluten-free chilli powder.

Freezing:
To reheat after freezing, simply defrost in the fridge, then warm through in the microwave or in a saucepan over a medium heat.

Curries are one of my most-loved recipes to make, and this lamb balti doesn't disappoint. It combines the perfect blend of spices with tender pieces of lamb. Serve this with my Indian roasted cauliflower pilau rice (page 256) for a tasty curry night for the whole family.

1. Put the lamb into a bowl with the yoghurt and mix to make sure all the meat is coated. Set aside.

2. Spray a frying pan with cooking oil, then add the onion and fry for a couple of minutes until translucent.

3. Add the garlic and ginger with a pinch of salt and fry for a further 30 seconds, then add the tomatoes and cook on a medium heat until the tomatoes break down into a sauce.

4. Add the spices and 1 teaspoon of salt and stir until paste-like.

5. Add the lamb pieces and cook, stirring, until they are all covered in the sauce and lightly browned.

6. Add the green chilli, peppers, passata, water, fresh coriander and sweetener, if using.

7. Bring to a bubble, then reduce the heat, cover and simmer for 40 minutes, until the lamb is tender.

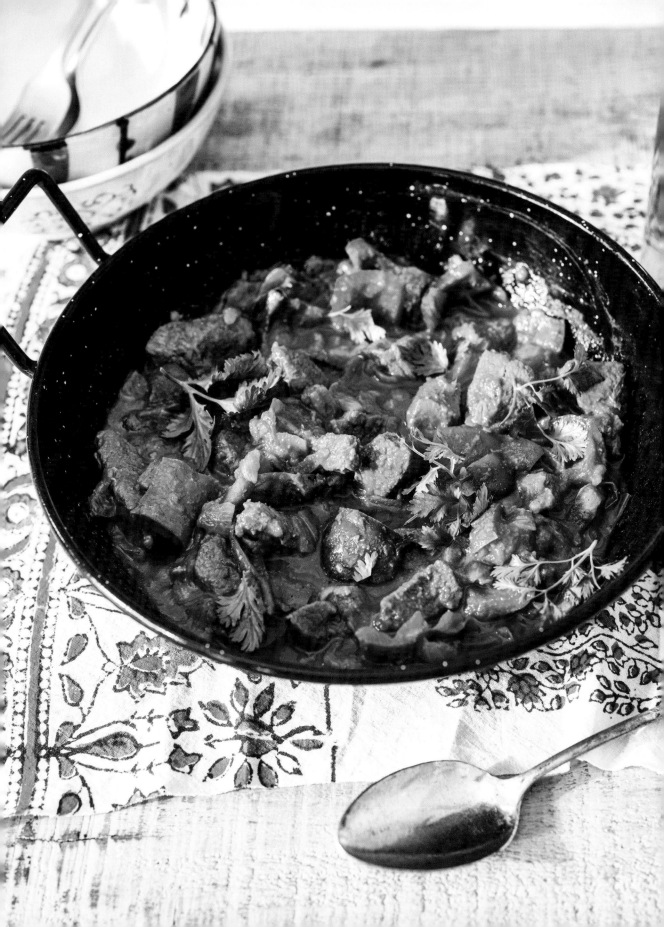

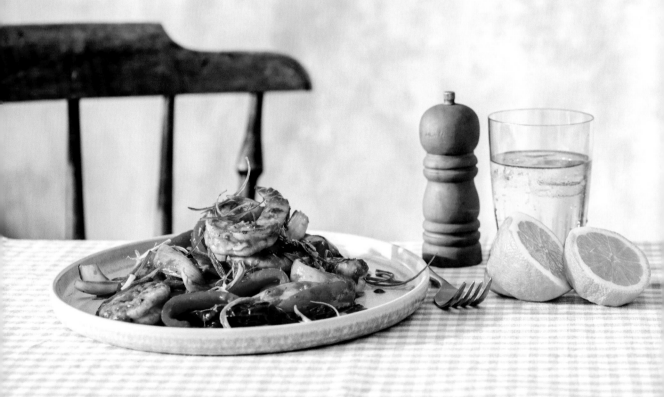

Fish and Seafood

Basil and Cherry Tomato
Cod Traybake

Creamy Tuscan
Halibut

Salmon Tikka
Traybake

Easy Prawn Laksa

Smoked Salmon
Poke Bowls

Bang Bang
Cod Bites

Szechuan Prawns
with Vegetables

Oven-baked
Salmon with Creamy
Butter Sauce

Coconut Fish
Curry

Tuna Melt
Sweet Potatoes

Easy Seafood
Paella

Basil and Cherry Tomato Cod Traybake

GF

DF

KCALS
196

FAT
6.9g

SAT FAT
1.1g

CARBS
6.1g

SUGARS
5.3g

FIBRE
2.5g

PROTEIN
26.2g

SALT
0.24g

SERVES 4

2 tablespoons extra
    virgin olive oil
4 garlic cloves, crushed
4 tablespoons finely
    chopped fresh basil
2 tablespoons lemon juice
40 cherry (or grape)
    tomatoes
250g (9oz) courgettes
    (zucchini), halved
    lengthways and sliced
4 fresh cod fillets (or other
    white fish of choice),
    approx. 140g (5oz) each
salt and freshly ground
    black pepper

Side suggestions:
Perfect with pasta, rice
or mashed potatoes.

Lower-carb side suggestions:
Cauliflower mash, or some
additional vegetables of
choice (asparagus, broccoli,
cauliflower, green beans, etc.).

**If you enjoy the flavours of pesto then this traybake is for you.
Gorgeous cod topped with a fresh basil marinade and baked in
the oven with tomatoes and courgettes for a simple, easy meal.**

1. Preheat the oven to 200°C/180°C fan/400°F/gas 6.

2. In a bowl combine the olive oil, garlic, basil and lemon juice.

3. Make 4 boats out of foil and place them on a baking tray.

4. Divide the tomatoes and courgettes between the foil boats.

5. Top each one with a piece of cod, then spoon over the basil sauce.

6. Season with salt and freshly ground black pepper.

7. Bake in the oven for 30–35 minutes, until the cod flakes easily
and the veg are softened.

8. Serve straight out of the oven with your favourite side.

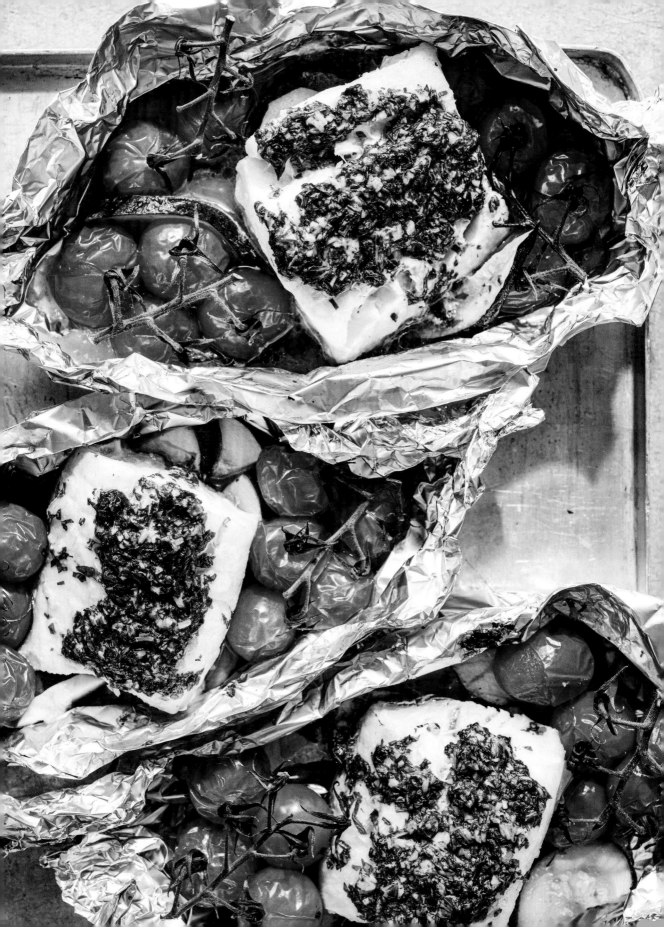

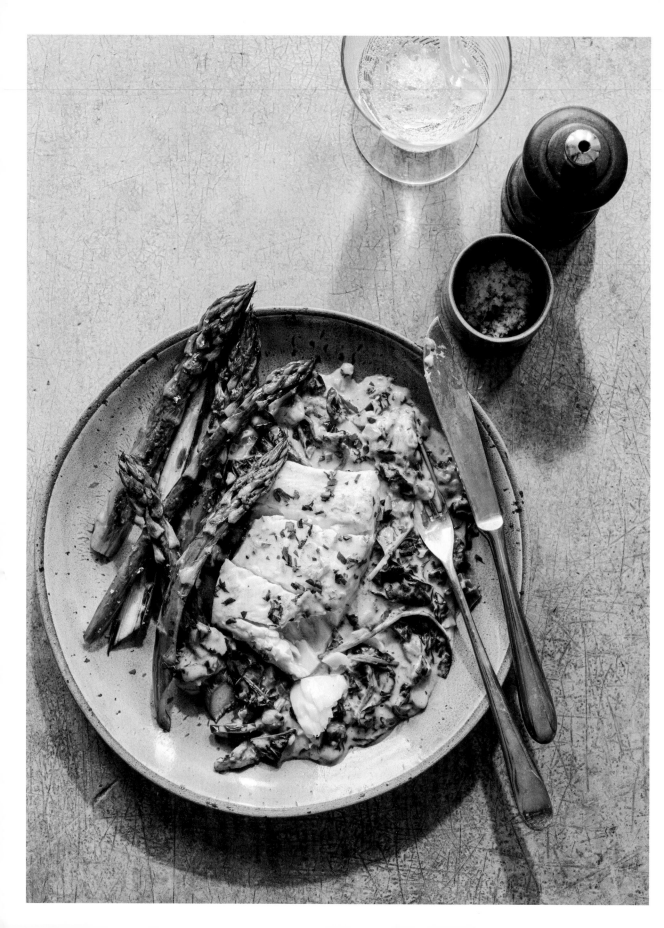

Creamy Tuscan Halibut

304
Calories

GF

SERVES 4

4 halibut fillets (or other white fish), approx. 140g (5oz) each
salt and freshly ground black pepper
olive oil spray
1 small onion, finely diced
360ml (12fl oz) chicken stock, plus an extra 125ml (4fl oz)
5 garlic cloves, crushed
50g (2oz) sun-dried tomatoes
½ tablespoon cornflour (cornstarch)
80g (3oz) cream cheese
120g (4oz) spinach, chopped
30g (1oz) Parmesan, grated
1 tablespoon chopped fresh parsley

Side suggestions:
This literally goes with anything you want. My personal favourites are pasta or mashed potatoes with an additional serving of green vegetables.

Lower-carb suggestion:
Cauliflower or celeriac (celery root) mash, roasted broccoli or roasted asparagus are a few of my faves.

Get ready to impress your taste buds with these halibut pieces in a garlicky Tuscan-inspired sauce made with sun-dried tomatoes and spinach. Best of all, it is ready and on the table in less than 30 minutes.

1. Season the fish with salt and freshly ground black pepper.

2. Heat a pan over a medium–high heat and spray it with olive oil. Add the fish and fry until lightly golden on both sides, then remove and set aside.

3. Spray the pan with a little more olive oil. Add the onion and fry until softened, adding a little of the extra stock to deglaze the pan of all the flavours from the fish.

4. Add the garlic and sun-dried tomatoes and keep adding the rest of the extra stock, reducing it down around the onion, garlic and sun-dried tomatoes until they are really softened and caramelized.

5. Mix the cornflour with a little water to make a slurry and add to the pan with the 360ml (12fl oz) of stock and the cream cheese. Bubble on a medium heat, stirring, until the cream cheese is all melted and the sauce has started to thicken, then add the spinach and Parmesan and stir until the spinach has wilted and the Parmesan has melted.

6. Put the halibut back into the pan and simmer on a low heat until it is cooked through (a couple of minutes).

7. Season with salt and freshly ground black pepper and sprinkle with the fresh parsley before serving.

KCALS
304

FAT
10.9g

SAT FAT
5.3g

CARBS
10.0g

SUGARS
6.4g

FIBRE
2.9g

PROTEIN
40.1g

SALT
1.24g

Salmon Tikka Traybake

SERVES 4

KCALS
335

FAT
16.0g

SAT FAT
3.0g

CARBS
13.4g

SUGARS
10.9g

FIBRE
4.5g

PROTEIN
32.1g

SALT
0.34g

4 tablespoons plain
  fat-free yoghurt
½ tablespoon grated
  fresh ginger
2 garlic cloves, crushed
1 teaspoon Kashmiri
  chilli powder
1 teaspoon paprika
¾ teaspoon turmeric
½ teaspoon ground cumin
½ teaspoon garam masala
½ teaspoon ground coriander
1 tablespoon fresh lemon
  juice
salt and freshly ground
  black pepper
500g (1lb 2oz) skinless
  salmon fillets, cubed
cooking oil spray
½ medium head of
  cauliflower, broken
  into florets
1 red pepper, sliced
1 green pepper, sliced
1 small red onion, sliced
a small handful of fresh
  coriander (cilantro),
  chopped

For the mint yoghurt:
125ml (4fl oz) plain fat-free
  yoghurt
1 tablespoon chopped
  fresh mint
1 tablespoon chopped
  fresh coriander (cilantro)
1 teaspoon lemon juice
1 teaspoon granulated
  sweetener (optional)

Gluten-free:
Use gluten-free chilli powder.

Forget chicken tikka – if you like salmon, then you will LOVE this salmon tikka traybake. Tender tikka-spiced coated salmon pieces are baked on one tray with peppers and cauliflower and paired with a fresh mint yoghurt.

1. In a bowl, combine the yoghurt, ginger, garlic, spices and lemon juice. Season with salt and freshly ground black pepper.

2. Add the salmon and leave to marinate for 30 minutes.

3. Preheat the oven to 230°C/210°C fan/450°F/gas 8.

4. Line a baking tray with parchment paper and spray the paper with cooking oil. Add the cauliflower, peppers and red onion and spray the top with cooking oil, then season with a pinch of salt.

5. Place in the oven and bake for 15 minutes.

6. Meanwhile, mix together the mint yoghurt ingredients.

7. Remove the tray from the oven and space out the vegetables evenly. Place the cubes of salmon between the vegetables, then spray with cooking oil. Reduce the oven to 200°C/180°C fan/400°F/gas 6 then bake for approx. 10 minutes, by which time the salmon should be cooked through.

8. Sprinkle with chopped fresh coriander and serve with the mint yoghurt. Perfect as it is, or you can serve with some rice.

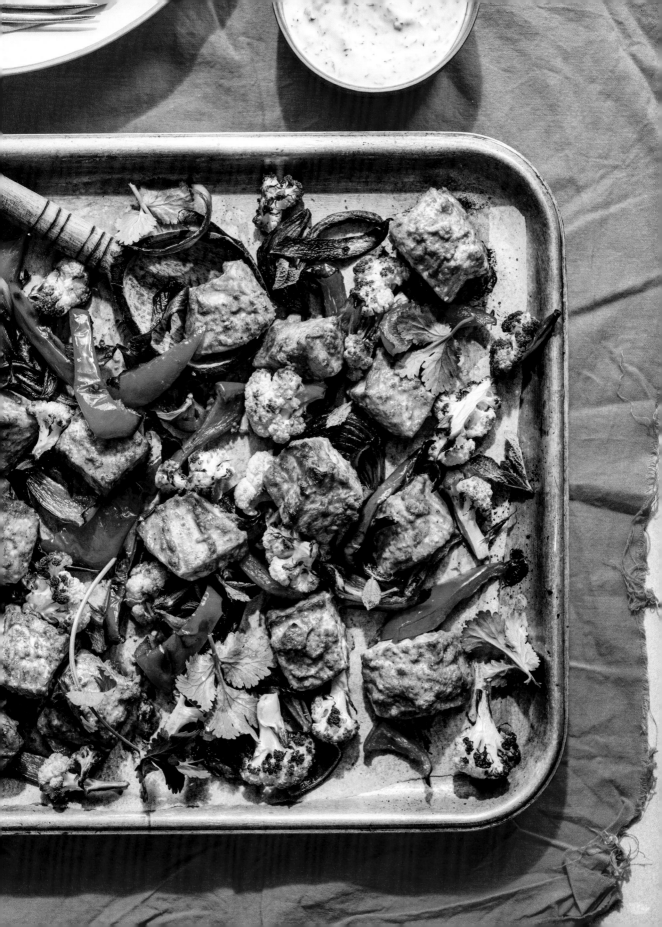

Easy Prawn Laksa

DF

KCALS
302

FAT
10.1g

SAT FAT
6.1g

CARBS
29.8g

SUGARS
5.7g

FIBRE
5.8g

PROTEIN
20.0g

SALT
2.95g

SERVES 4

For the paste:
1 small onion, chopped
2 garlic cloves, peeled
1 thumb-sized piece of
   fresh ginger, peeled
2–3 red chillies, deseeded
2 tablespoons curry powder
   (I used mild)
1 stalk of lemongrass (white
   part only), chopped
2 teaspoons tomato purée
   (paste)
pinch of salt
3 tablespoons water

For the laksa soup:
cooking oil spray
480ml (17fl oz) chicken stock
1 x 400ml (14fl oz) tin of light
   coconut milk
1 tablespoon fish sauce
½ tablespoon granulated
   sweetener (optional)
1 large carrot, halved, then
   sliced into thin sticks
100g (3½oz) beansprouts
12 mangetout (snow peas),
   halved
100g (3½oz) flat rice noodles
300g (10½oz) large raw
   prawns (shrimp)
salt and freshly ground
   black pepper

To serve:
2 spring onions (scallions),
   sliced (green part only)
handful of fresh coriander
   (cilantro), chopped

Gluten-free:
Use gluten-free curry
powder.

Two favourite ingredients, prawns (shrimp) and coconut milk, combine in this dreamy prawn laksa noodle soup, but it is so much more than soup – a simple but flavour-packed paste becomes a slurpable broth, packed with vegetables, prawns and rice noodles.

1. Put the ingredients for the paste into a mini food processor and pulse until they become a paste.

2. Place a deep frying pan over a medium–high heat and spray with some cooking oil, then add the paste and cook for a couple of minutes (watch that it doesn't burn). You can add a little of the stock if needed.

3. Add the stock, coconut milk, fish sauce, sweetener (if using), carrots, beansprouts and mangetout and simmer until the vegetables are tender.

4. Cook the noodles according to the package instructions.

5. Once the vegetables are tender, add the prawns and continue to cook until they are pink.

6. Add the cooked rice noodles and season with salt and freshly ground black pepper.

7. Serve sprinkled with chopped spring onions and coriander.

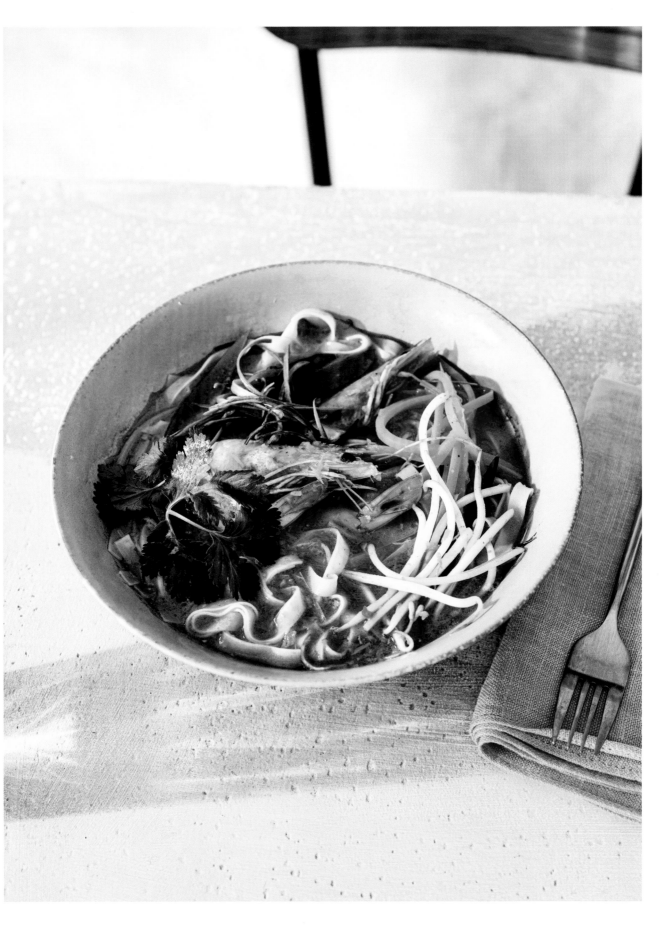

Smoked Salmon Poke Bowls

KCALS
489

FAT
20.4g

SAT FAT
3.4g

CARBS
49.6g

SUGARS
13.7g

FIBRE
6.0g

PROTEIN
23.7g

SALT
2.56g

SERVES 2

1 tablespoon reduced
   sodium soy sauce
½ tablespoon rice vinegar
1 teaspoon grated fresh ginger
½ tablespoon maple syrup
   (or honey)
½ teaspoon sesame oil
100g (3½oz) smoked salmon
80g (3oz) jasmine rice,
   rinsed
240ml (9fl oz) water
80g (3oz) frozen shelled
   edamame
salt
125g (4½oz) cucumber, diced
50g (2oz) avocado, diced
80g (3oz) julienned or
   grated carrot
chopped fresh coriander
   (cilantro)
black and white toasted
   sesame seeds
2 tablespoons light
   mayonnaise
2 tablespoons plain fat-free
   yoghurt
½ tablespoon sriracha

Gluten-free:
Use gluten-free soy sauce
and mayonnaise.

These are my go-to in the summer when I want a simple light meal. Diced smoked salmon (typically any sushi grade raw fish is used in poke bowls), is marinated and served over sticky white rice, with some edamame and vegetables, all drizzled with spicy sriracha mayo.

1. Whisk together the soy sauce, rice vinegar, ginger, maple syrup and sesame oil in a bowl. Add the smoked salmon and toss to coat. Refrigerate while you prepare everything else.

2. Put the rice into a saucepan with the water. Bring to the boil, simmer until the water is just absorbed, then cover the pan, turn off the heat and leave for 10 minutes.

3. Put the edamame into a bowl and cover with water. Put a plate on top and microwave for 4–5 minutes. Drain and season with a pinch of salt.

4. Build your bowl: in each bowl put some cucumber, avocado, carrot, edamame and coriander. Add the salmon and then the rice, adding a pinch of black and white toasted sesame seeds on top.

5. Mix together the mayo, yoghurt and sriracha and drizzle this over the top.

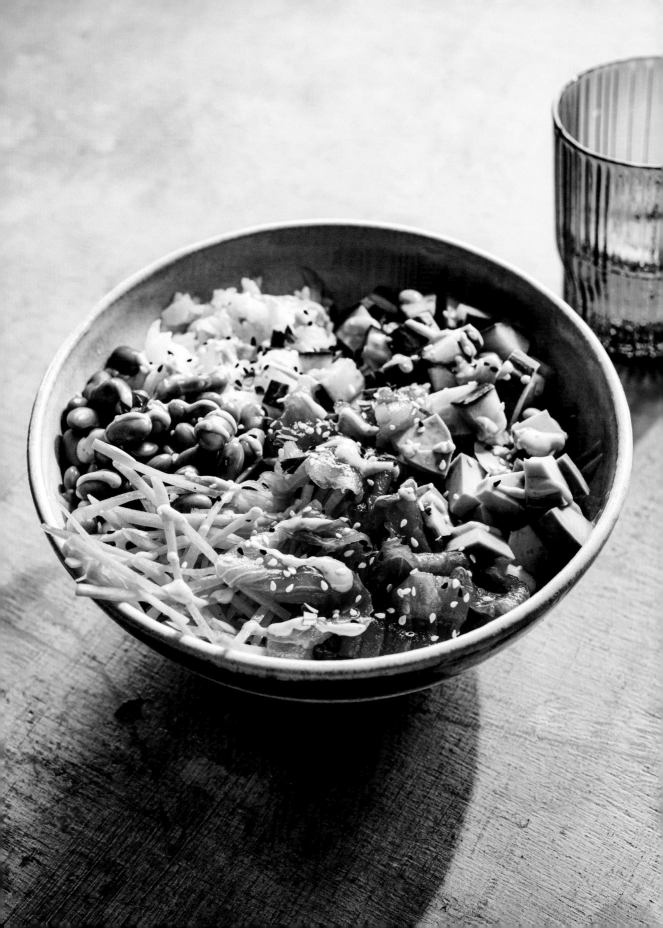

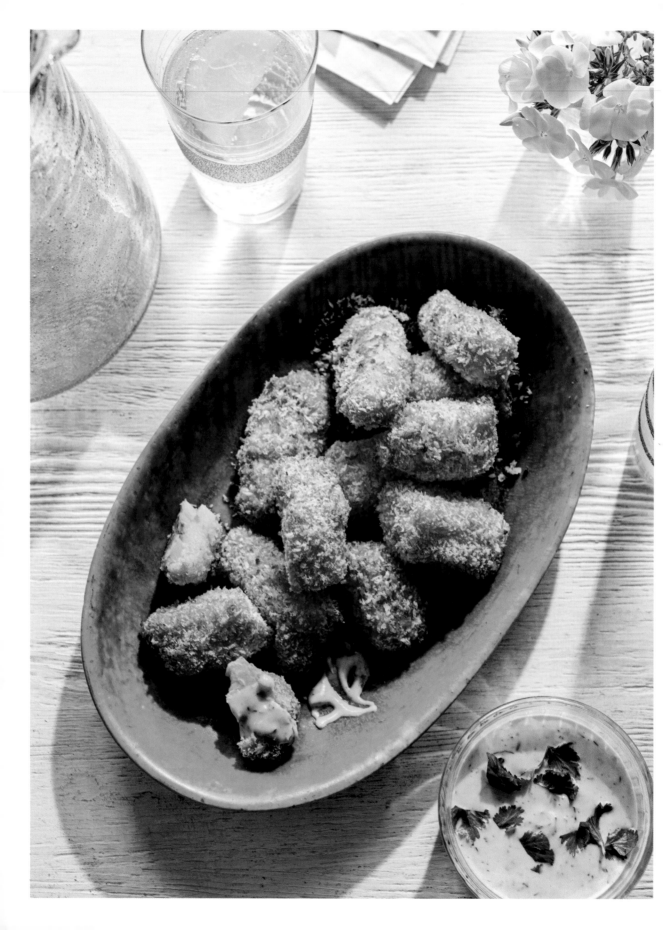

Bang Bang Cod Bites

199
Calories

SERVES 4

1 egg, beaten
½ teaspoon garlic powder
½ teaspoon onion powder
¼ teaspoon cayenne pepper
salt
450g (1lb) fresh cod,
    cut into bite-sized chunks
70g (2½oz) panko
    breadcrumbs
cooking oil spray
finely chopped fresh
    coriander (cilantro)

For the bang bang sauce:
2 tablespoons fat-free
    Greek yoghurt
2 tablespoons light
    mayonnaise
1 tablespoon sweet chilli
    sauce
1 teaspoon sriracha

These golden, panko-coated, oven-baked cod bites with a spicy sweet chilli mayo dip are very addictive. They work as a light lunch with some salad or as a filling main with some additional sides.

1. Preheat the oven to 230°C/210°C fan/450°F/gas 8.

2. Whisk the egg in a bowl with the garlic powder, onion powder, cayenne and a pinch of salt.

3. Pat the fish dry with kitchen paper.

4. Spread the panko on a plate.

5. Add the fish to the bowl of egg mixture and mix gently to fully coat.

6. Carefully roll the fish bites in the panko.

7. Line a baking sheet with parchment paper and spray the paper with cooking oil.

8. Add the cod bites to the tray and spray over the top with the cooking oil.

9. Bake in the oven for 12 minutes, until golden.

10. Meanwhile, mix the ingredients for the bang bang sauce together in a bowl.

11. Remove from the oven, sprinkle with fresh coriander and season with a pinch of salt and serve with the bang bang sauce.

KCALS
199

FAT
4.4g

SAT FAT
0.6g

CARBS
14.7g

SUGARS
2.1g

FIBRE
0.7g

PROTEIN
25.0g

SALT
0.72g

Szechuan Prawns with Vegetables

DF

KCALS
131

FAT
3.8g

SAT FAT
0.7g

CARBS
10.9g

SUGARS
4.7g

FIBRE
3.3g

PROTEIN
11.7g

SALT
2.34g

SERVES 4

cooking oil spray
1 onion, sliced
1 red pepper, sliced
2 garlic cloves, crushed
½ tablespoon grated
　fresh ginger
10 dried red chillies (use
　more or less, according to
　your desired spice level)
½ teaspoon crushed
　Szechuan peppercorns
250g (9oz) medium-sized
　raw prawns (shrimp)
2 tablespoons soy sauce
2 tablespoons hoisin sauce
2 tablespoons Shaoxing wine
　(or dry cooking sherry)
1 teaspoon sesame oil
125ml (4fl oz) water
1 tablespoon brown
　granulated sweetener
½ tablespoon cornflour
　(cornstarch)
2 spring onions (scallions),
　sliced

I love the spicy-sweet flavour of Szechuan-style sauce, and this recipe using large prawns and tender vegetables is a simple fakeaway to cook at home. Best of all, it's ready and on the table in less than 30 minutes.

1. Spray a frying pan with cooking oil.

2. Add the onion, red pepper, garlic, ginger and dried chillies and fry for a few minutes, until tender.

3. Add the Szechuan peppercorns and the prawns and fry until the prawns turn pink.

4. Add the soy sauce, hoisin sauce, Shaoxing wine, sesame oil, water and sweetener. Mix the cornflour with a little water to make a slurry and stir this in too. Simmer until the sauce thickens.

5. Sprinkle with sliced spring onions.

Note:
If you can't get Szechuan peppercorns, sub with regular freshly ground black pepper and a little lemon zest. It's worth sourcing some Shaoxing wine for that authentic flavour if you can (check local Chinese supermarkets), but dry sherry can be used in its place.

Lower-carb side suggestions:
Special fried cauliflower rice (page 239).

Gluten-free:
Use gluten-free soy sauce and hoisin sauce.

Vegetarian:
Swap the prawns for tofu or a meat substitute.

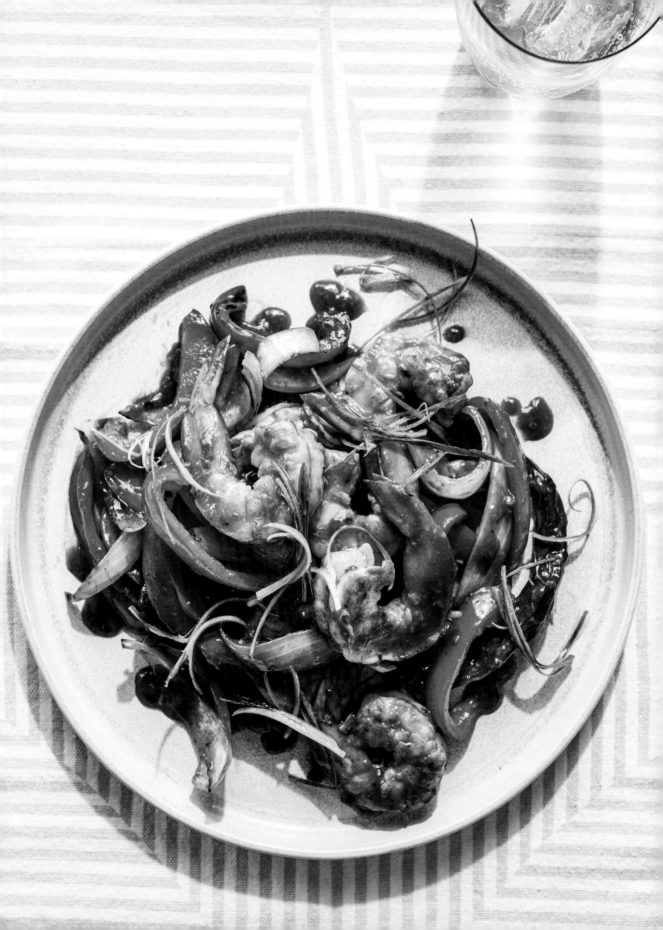

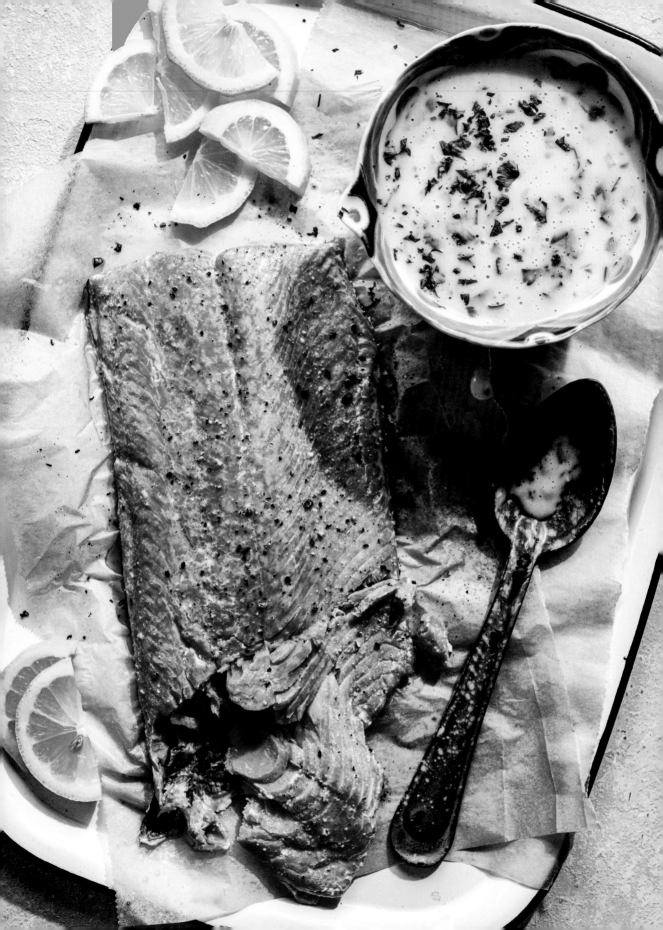

Oven-baked Salmon with Creamy Butter Sauce

SERVES 4

550g (1lb 4oz) piece of wild salmon fillet (or 4 pieces with a similar weight in total)
olive oil spray
salt and freshly ground black pepper

For the creamy butter sauce:
olive oil spray
1 shallot, finely diced
salt and freshly ground black pepper
2 tablespoons butter
3 tablespoons light cream cheese
240ml (9fl oz) fish or chicken stock
2 teaspoons cornflour (cornstarch)
1½ tablespoons chopped fresh parsley

Gluten-free:
Use gluten-free cornflour.

Side suggestion:
Great with some new potatoes cooked in stock and green veggies of your choice.

There's nothing quite like a tender oven-baked salmon with a creamy butter sauce to pour over the top, and this lighter creamy butter sauce definitely ticks all the boxes – it has slightly lower calories than a regular butter sauce but is definitely not lacking in flavour. It's a winning combination.

1. Preheat the oven to 220°C/200°C fan/425°F/gas 7.

2. Put the salmon on a baking tray lined with parchment paper, spray over the top with olive oil and season with salt and freshly ground black pepper.

3. Place in the oven and bake for 10–12 minutes. The time may vary depending on the thickness of fillet.

4. While the salmon is cooking, spray a small saucepan with olive oil, add the shallot and a pinch of salt and fry until lightly golden and translucent.

5. Add the butter and cream cheese and stir until melted and creamy, then add the stock. Mix the cornflour with a little water to make a slurry and stir this in in too, along with a pinch of freshly ground black pepper. Heat until the butter sauce is creamy and thickened (about 8 minutes), then stir in the parsley.

6. Serve the sauce with the salmon and a side of your choice.

GF

KCALS
345

FAT
23.2g

SAT FAT
7.4g

CARBS
3.5g

SUGARS
1.2g

FIBRE
0.6g

PROTEIN
30.2g

SALT
0.41g

Coconut Fish Curry

DF

KCALS
213

FAT
9.1g

SAT FAT
5.4g

CARBS
7.0g

SUGARS
4.8g

FIBRE
3.4g

PROTEIN
24.1g

SALT
0.32g

SERVES 4

455g (1lb) firm white fish
   (such as tilapia or halibut)
½ teaspoon turmeric
juice of ½ a lemon
pinch of salt

For the curry paste:
2 tablespoons tomato purée
   (paste)
1 teaspoon hot chilli powder
3 garlic cloves, crushed
1 thumb-sized piece of fresh
   ginger, peeled
2 teaspoons ground cumin
2 teaspoons ground coriander
1 teaspoon turmeric
60ml (2fl oz) water

For the curry:
cooking oil spray
1 onion, halved and
   thinly sliced
225ml (8fl oz) fish or
   chicken stock
175ml (6fl oz) light coconut
   milk
3 handfuls of spinach,
   chopped

Gluten-free:
Use gluten-free chilli powder.

Low-carb side:
Serve with cauliflower rice
(page 239).

This beautiful fish curry combines tender, flaky pieces of white fish with flavoursome spices from a simple homemade curry paste, all finished off with coconut milk for that creamy taste and spinach for some healthy greens.

1. Pat the fish dry, then put it into a ziplock bag with the turmeric, lemon juice and a pinch of salt and move it around in the bag to coat.

2. Put the paste ingredients into a mini food processor and pulse to a paste.

3. Place a frying pan (skillet) over a medium–high heat and spray with cooking oil, then add the onion and fry until lightly golden and softened.

4. Add the paste and cook for a further couple of minutes, being careful not to let it burn, and adding a little more water if needed.

5. Add the stock and coconut milk, then carefully add the fish. Bring to the boil, then cover and simmer for 8–10 minutes until the fish is cooked.

6. Add the chopped spinach to the pan and stir gently until wilted.

7. Taste and season with salt if needed.

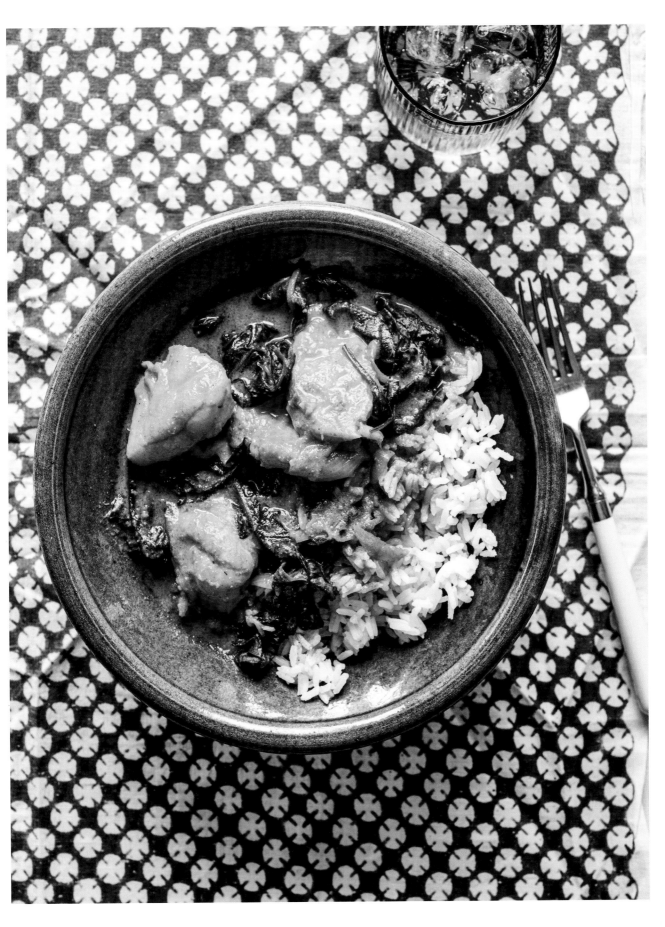

Tuna Melt Sweet Potatoes

SERVES 4

2 large sweet potatoes
(350g/12½oz each)
cooking oil spray
salt and freshly ground
black pepper
1 x 200g (7oz) tin of tuna,
drained
2 tablespoons light
mayonnaise
3 tablespoons fat-free
Greek yoghurt
½ a small red pepper,
finely diced
1 stalk of celery, finely diced
1 garlic clove, crushed
3 spring onions (scallions),
finely chopped
6 pickle slices, finely chopped
(and a little pickle juice)
60g (2oz) Cheddar or Red
Leicester, grated
chopped fresh chives or
spring onions (scallions),
to serve

Gluten-free:
Use gluten-free mayonnaise.

Note:
The cooking time for sweet
potatoes may vary if bigger
or smaller in size.

KCALS
325

FAT
9.3g

SAT FAT
4.0g

CARBS
38.2g

SUGARS
20.9g

FIBRE
6.7g

PROTEIN
18.7g

SALT
1.16g

My family are big on baked sweet potatoes and we also love tuna melts, so what could be better than these tuna melt sweet potatoes? The perfect tuna mayo salad is piled high over warming baked sweet potatoes, topped with cheese and baked to a melting heavenly goodness.

1. Pierce the sweet potatoes. You can either cook them in the microwave or in the oven.

For the microwave (1000 wattage): place in the microwave and microwave for 3 minutes. Turn them over and microwave for an additional 3 minutes (if your sweet potatoes are slightly smaller or bigger, you may need to adjust the time).

For the oven (for crispier skin): Preheat the oven to 220°C/200°C fan/425°F/gas 7. Spray the skin with cooking oil and rub in a little salt. Place on a baking tray lined with foil and bake for approx. 45–50 minutes. The sweet potatoes should feel soft inside when pierced with a knife or fork, and should have a slightly crisp skin.

2. Once the sweet potatoes are cooked, allow them to cool slightly, then slice them in half and scoop out some of the flesh, so you have 4 sweet potato boats.

3. Put the sweet potato flesh into a bowl with the tuna, mayo, Greek yoghurt, red pepper, celery, garlic, spring onions, pickles (plus 1–2 tablespoons of pickle juice) and a pinch of salt and freshly ground black pepper, and fold together until combined.

4. Season the sweet potato boats with salt and freshly ground black pepper, then spoon the tuna salad into the boats. Top with the grated cheese, place on a baking tray and bake at 220°C/200°C fan/425°F/gas 7 for approx. 10–15 minutes, until the cheese is melted and golden.

5. Sprinkle with chopped chives or spring onions and serve with a mixed salad.

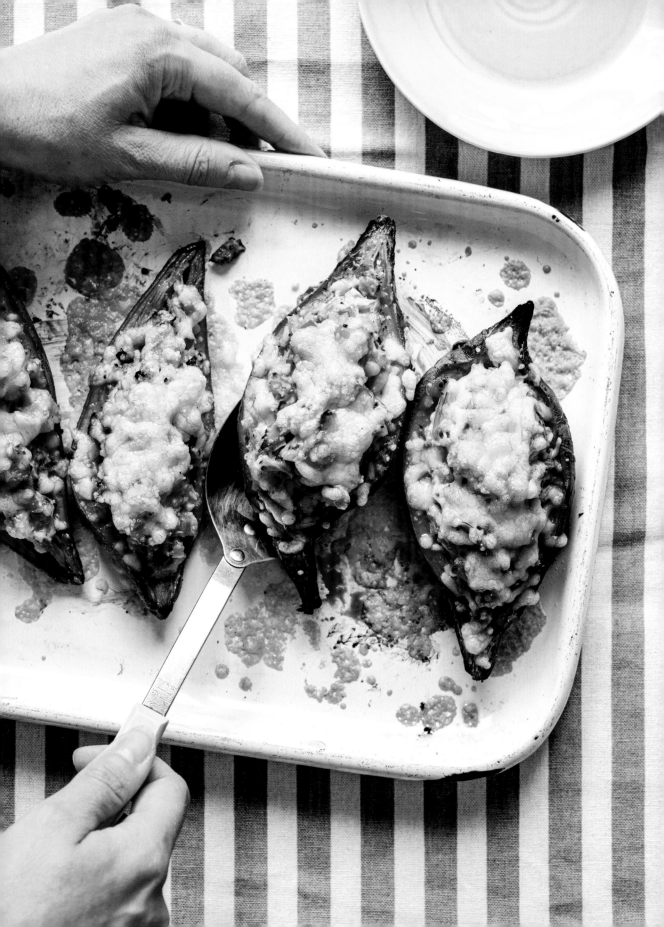

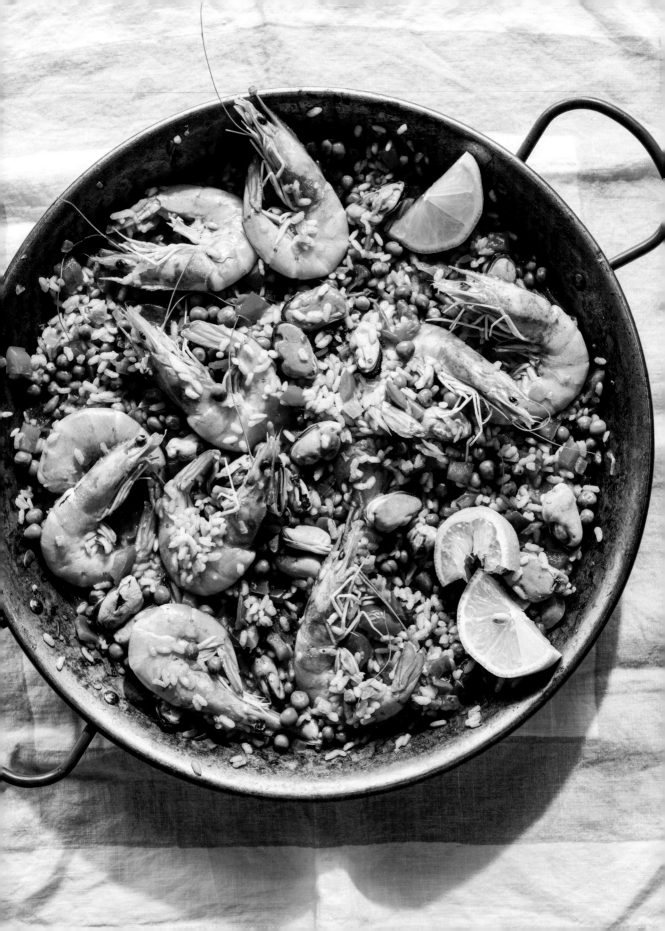

Easy Seafood Paella

SERVES 4

1 tablespoon extra virgin
   olive oil
1 large onion, finely diced
½ red pepper, finely diced
½ green pepper, finely diced
3 garlic cloves, crushed
10 cherry tomatoes, quartered
pinch of saffron, soaked in
   2 tablespoons hot water
   (soak well in advance if
   you can)
1 teaspoon paprika
pinch of red chilli flakes
salt and freshly ground
   black pepper
200g (7oz) paella rice (or
   other short-grain rice),
   rinsed
100g (3½oz) frozen peas
600ml (20fl oz) chicken
   stock
20 large shell-on prawns
   (shrimp)
200g (7oz) cooked mussels
   (I use ones that are not in
   shells, but you can also use
   fresh mussels)
small handful of fresh
   parsley, chopped
1 lemon, cut into wedges

Paella doesn't need to be complicated if you use this simple, easy recipe. Fragrant saffron rice with vegetables and seafood – everyone will love digging into this dish. Occasionally when I can't get shell-on prawns I'll use a frozen seafood mix, and it works well.

1. Heat the olive oil in a large frying pan or paella pan and fry the onion until softened and caramelized.

2. Add the peppers and garlic and fry for a couple of minutes until softened.

3. Add the tomatoes, saffron (with its soaking water), paprika, red chilli flakes and a good pinch of salt and freshly ground black pepper. Cook until the tomatoes are slightly softened and the water from the saffron has evaporated.

4. Add the rice and give a gentle stir just to combine everything.

5. Add the peas and pour in the stock (do not stir again).

6. Bring to the boil, then reduce the heat and simmer uncovered for 10 minutes.

7. Add the prawns and mussels, nestling some of them into the rice, and continue to simmer until the liquid has been absorbed (approx. a further 2–5 minutes).

8. Once all the liquid is absorbed, put a lid on the pan, turn off the heat and leave for 12–15 minutes (the steam trapped underneath will continue to cook the paella).

9. Sprinkle with fresh parsley and garnish with lemon wedges.

364 Calories

GF

DF

KCALS
364

FAT
5.5g

SAT FAT
1.0g

CARBS
50.9g

SUGARS
7.6g

FIBRE
5.5g

PROTEIN
25.1g

SALT
2.0g

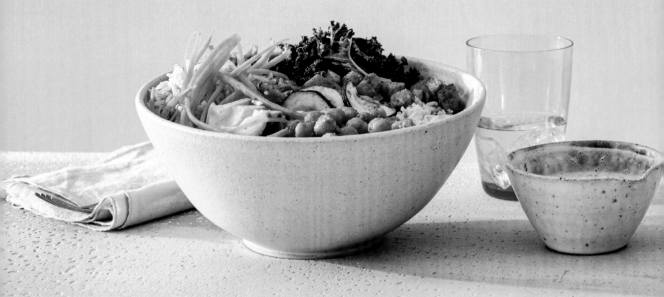

Vegetarian

Pizza Calzones

Honey and Garlic
Tofu Stir-fry

Mushroom
Carnitas Bowl

Lemon, Garlic, Cauliflower
and Courgette Pasta

Creamy Sweetcorn
and Leek Risotto

Garlic Mushroom,
Onion and Jalapeño
Filo Tart

Easy Indian Paneer
Stir-fry

Peanut Lentil Curry

Chickpea, Tomato
and Feta Traybake

Chickpea Sweet
Potato Buddha Bowls

Butternut Squash
and Ricotta Bake

Sweet Potato and
Kidney Bean Burgers
with Curried Dip

Taco Veggie
Pasta Bake

Pizza Calzones

KCALS
272

FAT
10.5g

SAT FAT
6.0g

CARBS
27.6g

SUGARS
3.7g

FIBRE
2.1g

PROTEIN
15.7g

SALT
0.96g

MAKES 6 CALZONES

180g (6oz) plain (all-purpose) flour, plus 1 tablespoon set aside for dusting
2 teaspoons baking powder
salt
200g (7oz) fat-free Greek yoghurt
1 large egg
½ teaspoon garlic powder
130g (4½oz) Cheddar, sliced
30g (1oz) Parmesan or vegetarian Italian-style hard cheese, grated
olive oil spray

For the pizza sauce:
120g (4oz) passata
4 tablespoons tomato purée (paste)
½ teaspoon onion powder
½ teaspoon garlic powder
1 teaspoon dried basil
1 teaspoon dried oregano
pinch of granulated sweetener

Variations:
Try adding other fillings like veggies, olives, etc. Or if not vegetarian, you can add pepperoni, ham and pineapple, or chicken, with some barbecue sauce instead of the pizza sauce. Be careful not to over-fill the calzones, otherwise they may burst open.

This is a serious pizza treat for the weekend – no-one can resist these calzone delights. Great for picnics in the summer too. Serve them just as they are with some salad, or add your choice of sides for the ultimate fakeaway meal.

1. Preheat the oven to 200°C/180°C fan/400°F/gas 6.

2. Mix the ingredients for the pizza sauce together in a bowl.

3. In a bowl combine the flour with the baking powder and a pinch of salt.

4. Add the yoghurt to the bowl and use a wooden spoon or spatula to mix the ingredients together. As the dough starts to come together, use your hands to knead it into a ball until the sides of the bowl are clean.

5. Divide the dough into 6 equal-sized balls.

6. Dust a surface with flour, then add one ball of the dough and lightly dust over the top with flour. Place a square of parchment paper on top of the ball and flatten down with a heavy saucepan, then roll flat (rotating and flipping the dough as you roll) until you have a rough oval shape about 15 x 20cm (6 x 8 inches).

7. Transfer to a baking tray lined with parchment paper.

8. Beat the egg in a bowl with the garlic powder.

9. Add some pizza sauce and Cheddar to one half of the dough and brush around the edge with the egg wash. Fold over and crimp together with a fork.

10. Repeat with the other 5 balls.

11. Brush over the tops of the calzones with the egg wash, ensuring you cover them completely. Sprinkle with the Parmesan and a pinch of salt.

12. Spray over the tops of the calzones with olive oil.

13. Bake in the oven for 20 minutes, until golden.

14. Enjoy!

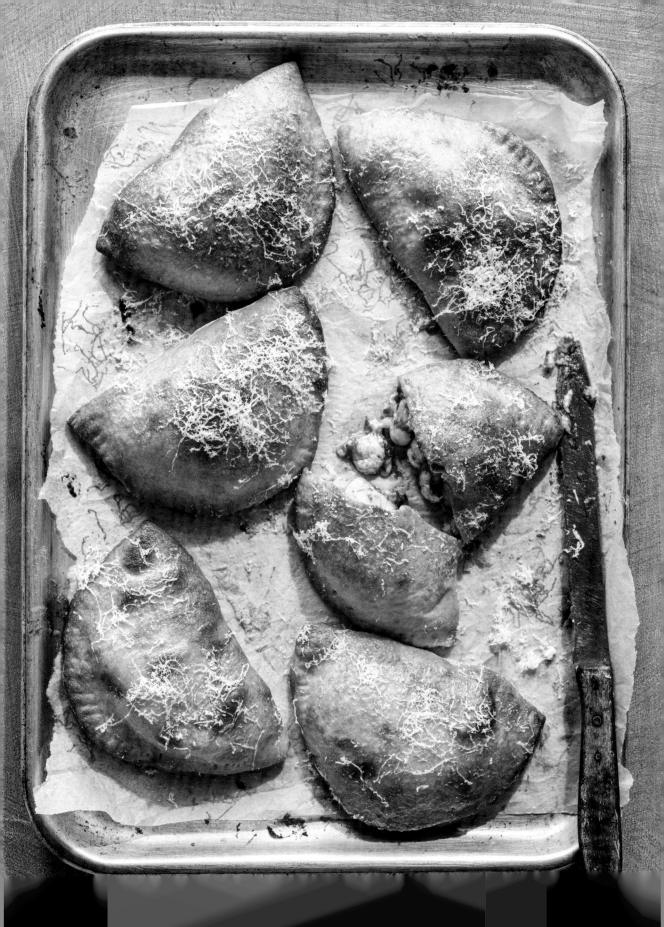

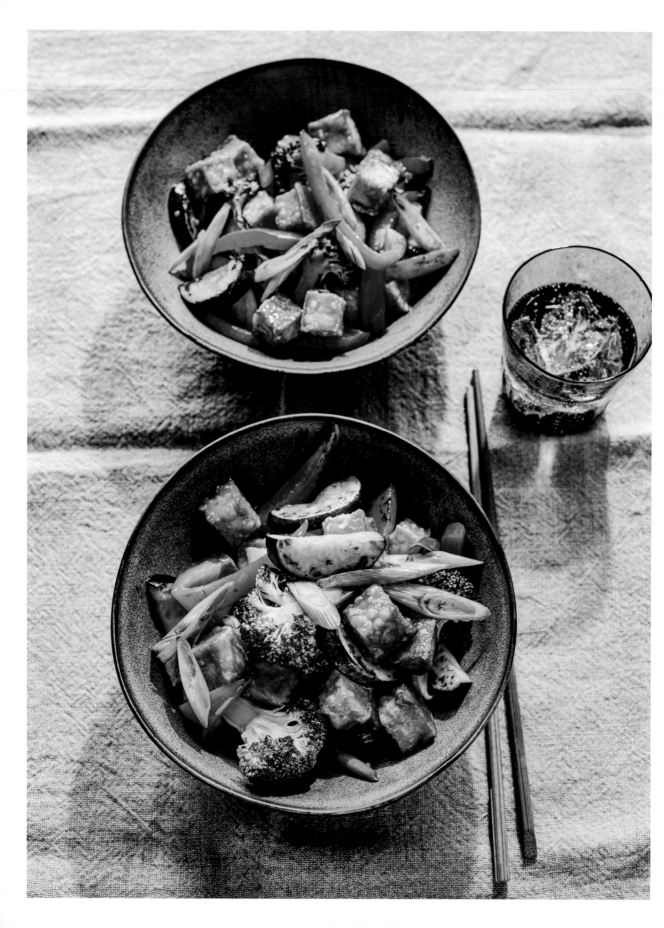

Honey and Garlic Tofu Stir-fry

270
Calories

V

DF

SERVES 4

For the crispy tofu:
400g (14oz) extra firm tofu
½ teaspoon garlic powder
½ tablespoon soy sauce
1 tablespoon cornflour
  (cornstarch)
cooking oil spray

For the stir-fry:
200g (7oz) broccoli florets
150g (5½oz) courgettes
  (zucchini), halved and
  chopped
1 red pepper, chopped
150g (5½oz) carrots, halved
  lengthways and sliced
5 garlic cloves, crushed
4 spring onions (scallions),
  sliced

For the sauce:
3 tablespoons honey
3 tablespoons soy sauce
  (low sodium if you prefer)
120ml (4fl oz) water
¾ tablespoon cornflour
  (cornstarch)

Gluten-free:
Use gluten-free soy sauce
and cornflour.

Low-carb side suggestion:
Serve over cauliflower rice
(page 239) or sautéed
vegetable noodles.

Not vegetarian?:
Feel free to swap the tofu
for a protein of your choice
– chicken, pork, prawns
(shrimp), etc.

Who needs take-out when you can make this quick takeaway dish at home – crispy tofu pieces and tender vegetables, all finished off with my super easy but flavoursome honey garlic sauce? Many people are wary of eating tofu, and I was too until I was introduced to the method of baking it until crispy in the oven, then tossing it in a sauce. If you've tried tofu and hated it, I challenge you to try this dish. I am sure most of you will be converted.

1. Drain the tofu, place between sheets of kitchen paper or inside a clean kitchen towel, then place a heavy item on top and leave for about 15 minutes for the excess liquid to drain off.

2. Preheat the oven to 200°C/180°C fan/400°F/gas 6.

3. Cut the tofu into 2cm (¾ inch) cubes. Put them into a bowl with the garlic powder and soy sauce and toss to coat. Then sprinkle with the cornflour and toss again.

4. Line a tray with parchment paper and spray the paper with cooking oil. Add the tofu cubes and spread out evenly, making sure they are not touching each other. Spray over the top with cooking oil.

5. Bake for 30 minutes until golden and crispy (I rotate the tray halfway). Remove from the oven and set aside.

6. Spray a frying pan or wok with cooking oil. Add the broccoli, courgettes, red pepper, carrots and garlic and stir-fry until tender.

7. Whisk together all the sauce ingredients in a bowl. Add to the pan and let it bubble until it thickens, then add the tofu and toss until everything is coated in the sauce and heated through.

8. Sprinkle with sliced spring onions and serve.

KCALS
270

FAT
8.1g

SAT FAT
1.4g

CARBS
28.1g

SUGARS
19.7g

FIBRE
7.2g

PROTEIN
17.5g

SALT
1.88g

428
Calories

Mushroom Carnitas Bowl

KCALS
428

FAT
9.4g

SAT FAT
1.8g

CARBS
61.8g

SUGARS
14.1g

FIBRE
12.8g

PROTEIN
17.8g

SALT
1.92g

SERVES 2

For the mushroom carnitas:
300g (10½oz) mushrooms
   (large portobello cap), gills
   removed, shredded
1 garlic clove, crushed
80g (3oz) onions, halved
   and thinly sliced
4 tablespoons freshly
   squeezed orange juice
1 tablespoons lime juice
60ml (2fl oz) vegetable stock
pinch of cayenne pepper
1 teaspoon ground cumin
1 teaspoon paprika
pinch of salt
pinch of freshly ground
   black pepper
½ teaspoon dried oregano
olive oil spray

For the pico de gallo:
125g (4½oz) tomatoes,
   diced
50g (2oz) onion, finely
   chopped
½ large jalapeño, deseeded
   and diced
1 tablespoon finely chopped
   coriander (cilantro)
¼ teaspoon salt
pinch of freshly ground
   black pepper
2 teaspoons lime juice

To serve:
Fresh coriander (cilantro),
   chopped
2 servings of lime coriander
   rice (see page 122)
6 tablespoons tinned
   black beans
6 tablespoons tinned
   sweetcorn, warmed
60g (2oz) avocado, mashed
125g (4½oz) romaine lettuce
grated Cheddar (optional)

Carnitas is one of my favourite Mexican dishes. It is usually made with tender slow-cooked meat that is pulled apart and then crisped on the edges, all seasoned with delicious spices. In this recipe I use thinly shredded portobello mushrooms to create a vegetarian-friendly version. The part my family love most about carnitas is choosing what toppings to pair with it. In this recipe I pair it with a homemade pico de gallo, lime coriander rice and some other yummy sides, but you really can add any toppings you like.

1. Preheat the oven to 230°C/210°C fan/450°F/gas 8.

2. Put all the ingredients for the mushroom carnitas on a baking tray and toss to combine. Spray over the top with olive oil.

3. Bake for 20–25 minutes, flipping halfway, then put under a hot grill (broiler) for 8 minutes until crispy on the edges. Sprinkle with chopped coriander.

4. Cook the lime coriander rice.

5. Mix the pico de gallo ingredients and place in the fridge until ready to eat (or you can make it the night before for best flavour). You could also use another salsa of your choice.

6. Build your bowl with mushrooms, rice, pico de gallo.

7. Serve with the black beans, sweetcorn, avocado and lettuce, and enjoy!

Lower-carb suggestions:
Omit the rice, and serve with cauliflower rice (page 239) or roasted butternut squash cubes.

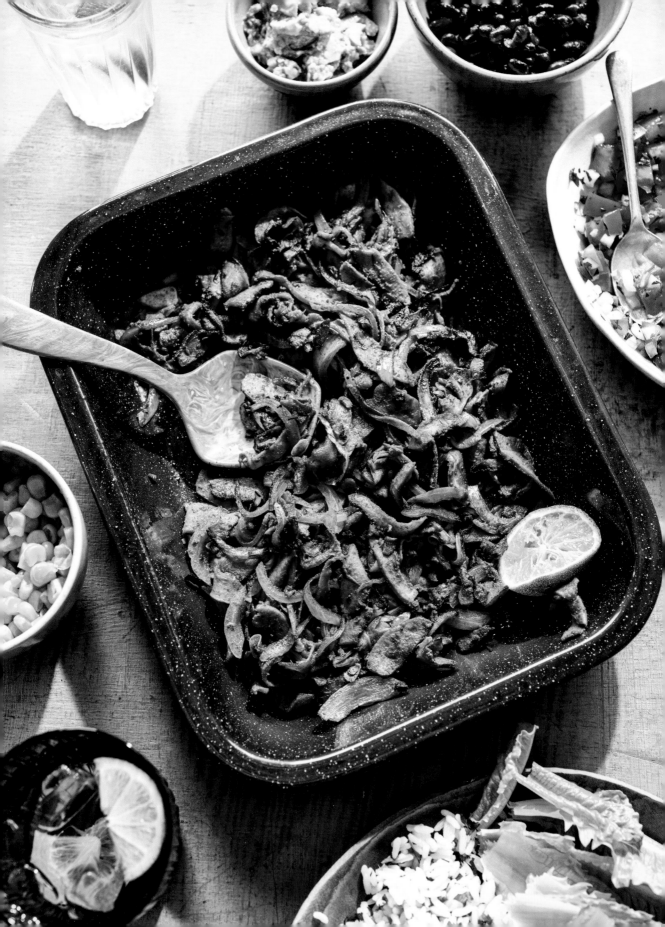

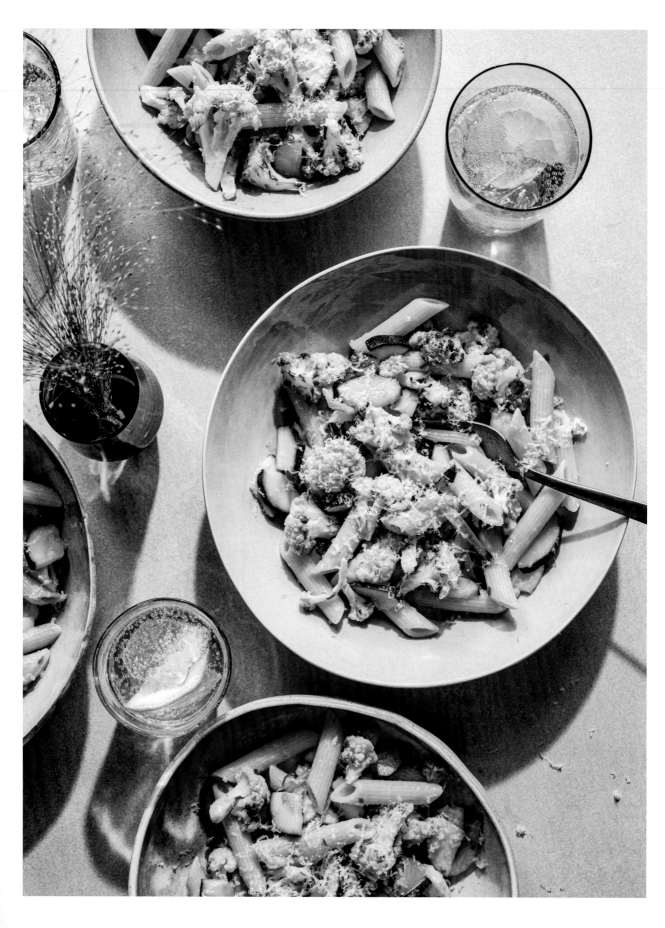

Lemon, Garlic, Cauliflower and Courgette Pasta

SERVES 4

olive oil spray
1 head of cauliflower, broken into small florets
1 small onion, thinly sliced
salt and freshly ground black pepper
250g (9oz) dried penne pasta (or any pasta you like)
½ tablespoon extra virgin olive oil
½ tablespoon butter
6 garlic cloves, crushed
pinch of red chilli flakes
240ml (9fl oz) vegetable stock
200g (7oz) courgette (zucchini), halved and sliced
juice and zest of 1 small lemon
2 tablespoons chopped fresh parsley

Optional:
Add some grated Parmesan or vegetarian Italian-style hard cheese. If not vegetarian, some cooked chicken or prawns are a great addition to this recipe too.

Dairy-free:
Use all olive oil instead of half oil and half butter.

Gluten-free:
Use gluten-free pasta.

Many pasta dishes have tomatoes as the main hero of the sauce, but this combination of lemon and garlic with herbs and vegetables makes an amazingly fresh, light and tangy sauce. Fab just as it is, or with some added protein of your choice.

1. Preheat the oven to 220°C/200°C fan/425°F/gas 7. Line a large baking tray with parchment paper and spray with olive oil.

2. Put the cauliflower and onion on the lined tray, season with salt and freshly ground black pepper, and roast for 25–30 minutes, until lightly browned on the edges.

3. Cook the pasta according to the package instructions, then drain, reserving about half a cup of the cooking water.

4. Heat the oil and butter in a frying pan or wok. Add the garlic and chilli flakes and cook until softened and golden.

5. Gradually add the stock, reducing it down until just a small amount remains in the pan, then add the courgettes and simmer for a couple of minutes.

6. Add the roasted cauliflower, cooked pasta, lemon juice, lemon zest, reserved pasta water and fresh parsley, and toss until combined.

7. Taste and season with salt and freshly ground black pepper.

KCALS
331

FAT
4.8g

SAT FAT
1.3g

CARBS
54.9g

SUGARS
7.8g

FIBRE
7.7g

PROTEIN
13.2g

SALT
0.21g

Creamy Sweetcorn and Leek Risotto

316
Calories

V

DF

GF

KCALS
316

FAT
4.6g

SAT FAT
2.4g

CARBS
57.8g

SUGARS
5.4g

FIBRE
5.9g

PROTEIN
7.9g

SALT
0.94g

SERVES 4

1.5 litres (2½ pints) vegetable
   stock
olive oil spray
2 leeks, trimmed, thinly sliced
   (200g/7oz) and washed
1 tablespoon white wine
   vinegar
250g (9oz) arborio rice
240g (8½oz) frozen
   sweetcorn
60ml (2fl oz) coconut milk
salt and freshly ground
   black pepper

Variations:

Add some curry powder
or chilli flakes for a spicy
alternative.

Sweetcorn and leeks make a beautiful pair in this creamy
dairy-free risotto that uses puréed sweetcorn and coconut
milk for that decadent creamy risotto taste. A simple recipe
that you can easily adapt every time you make it.

1. Put the stock into a small saucepan and keep warm on
a medium heat.

2. Spray a large frying pan with olive oil, then add the leeks
and fry until softened.

3. Add the white wine vinegar and cook until it evaporates.

4. Add the rice and fry until it just starts to go translucent.

5. Add half the sweetcorn, then gradually start adding the stock,
a large ladle at a time, stirring until it reduces down before
adding more, reserving a little of the stock.

6. When the rice is cooked and tender (about 30–35 minutes),
blend the rest of the sweetcorn with the reserved stock to make
a purée. Stir this into the risotto with the coconut milk until silky
and creamy.

7. Season with salt and freshly ground black pepper.

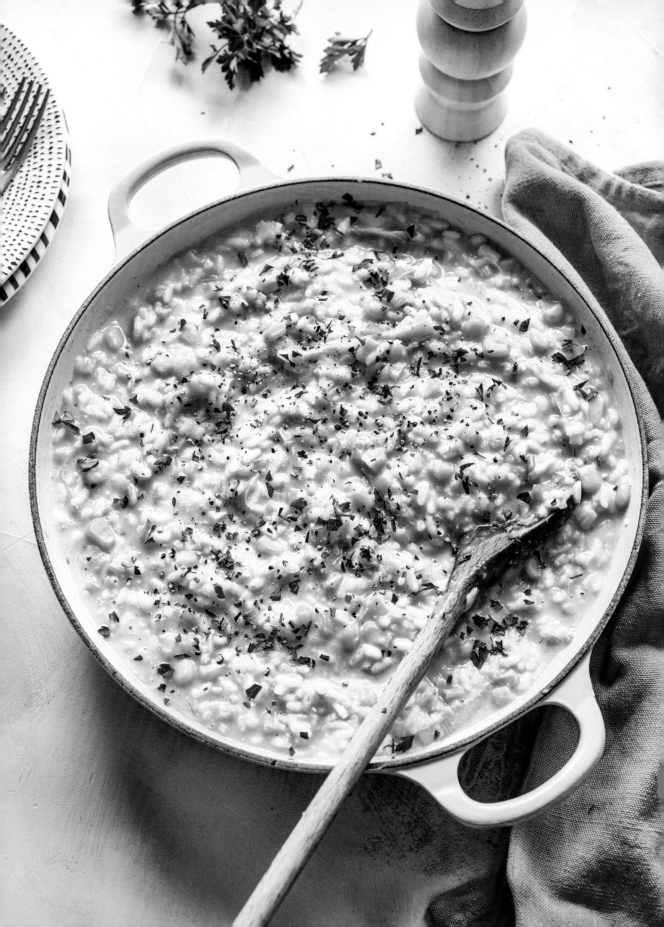

Garlic Mushroom, Onion and Jalapeño Filo Tart

KCALS
264

FAT
12.0g

SAT FAT
6.0g

CARBS
24.2g

SUGARS
2.4g

FIBRE
3.6g

PROTEIN
13.5g

SALT
0.93g

SERVES 4

cooking oil spray
1 small onion, halved and
    sliced
300g (10½oz) cremini
    mushrooms, sliced
2 garlic cloves, crushed
120ml (4fl oz) vegetable
    stock
4 sheets of filo pastry
1 egg, beaten
100g (3½oz) mature
    Cheddar, grated
1–2 jalapeños, thinly sliced
salt and freshly ground
    black pepper
chopped fresh chives

Side suggestions:
A simple mixed salad of
baby leaves with a light
dressing of your choice.

This yummy tart, made with light filo pastry and topped with sautéed garlic mushrooms, onions and slices of jalapeño for a spicy kick is such a simple recipe but packed with flavour. Good for a light lunch with a salad or can even be enjoyed as a main.

1. Preheat the oven to 180°C/160°C fan/350°F/gas 4.

2. Place a frying pan over a medium–high heat and spray it with cooking oil. Add the onion, mushrooms and garlic and fry for a couple of minutes until lightly golden, then start adding a little bit of stock at a time and reducing it down around the mushrooms and onions, repeating until all the stock has been absorbed and the mushrooms and onions are lovely and caramelized. Set aside.

3. Line a 33 x 24cm (13 x 9½inch) baking tray with parchment paper and spray the paper with cooking oil.

4. Lay the 4 sheets of filo on the baking tray, one on top of the other. Then roughly fold over the edges to make a large rectangular shape.

5. Spray the top with more cooking oil and bake in the oven for about 6–8 minutes, just until lightly golden.

6. Remove from the oven and carefully brush the pastry case with the beaten egg.

7. Add the mushroom and onion mixture to the tart case in an even layer. Top with the Cheddar, and scatter the jalapeño slices on top. Season with a little pinch of salt and freshly ground black pepper.

8. Put back into the oven and bake for about 10–15 minutes, until the cheese is all melted and golden.

9. Sprinkle with fresh chopped chives, then slice and serve.

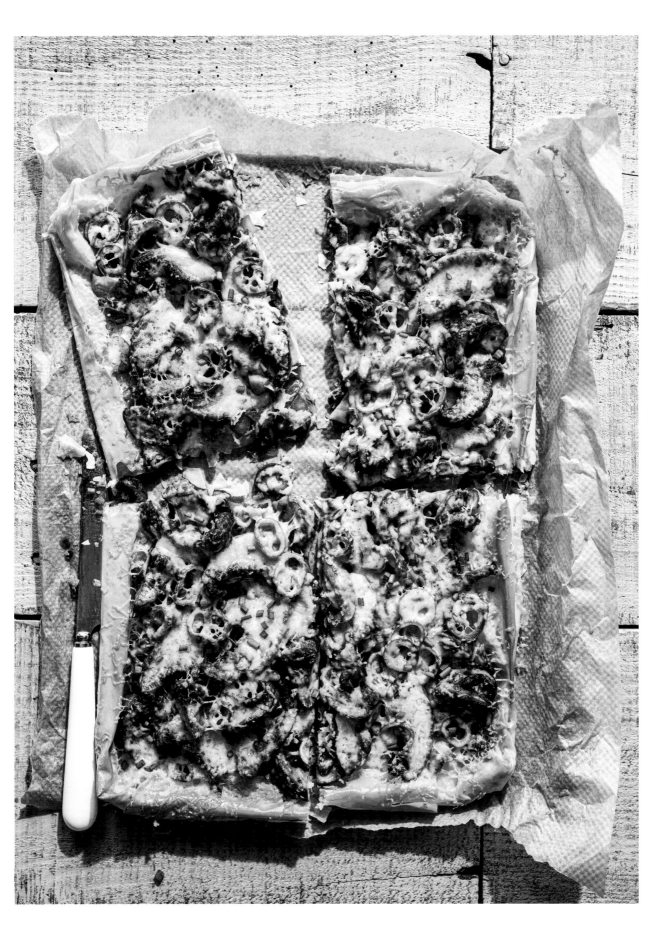

Easy Indian Paneer Stir-fry

SERVES 4

1 tablespoon ghee (or oil of choice)
300g (10½oz) Indian paneer cheese, cut into cubes
salt
1 teaspoon cumin seeds
1 small onion, diced
2 garlic cloves, crushed
½ tablespoon grated fresh ginger
200g (7oz) cauliflower florets
1 red pepper, chopped
1 green pepper, chopped
150g (5½oz) carrots, sliced thinly
1 courgette (zucchini), halved and sliced
1–2 red chillies, sliced (or a pinch of red chilli flakes)
120ml (4fl oz) vegetable stock
80g (3oz) frozen peas
2 tablespoons medium curry powder
juice of ½ a lemon
chopped fresh coriander (cilantro), optional

KCALS
372

FAT
23.5g

SAT FAT
13.9g

CARBS
13.3g

SUGARS
9.6g

FIBRE
7.2g

PROTEIN
23.3g

SALT
0.21g

Sides:
We love this just as it is, but you can also serve it with rice or as a side to other Indian dishes.

Gluten-free:
Use gluten-free curry powder.

When it comes to Indian dishes, one ingredient I champion is paneer cheese. It's a great vegetarian ingredient for curries, and regularly features on my menu when I fancy an Indian-inspired meat-free dish. This easy stir-fry combines golden cubes of paneer with tender stir-fried vegetables, all seasoned with beautiful Indian spices.

1. Heat half the ghee or oil in a deep frying pan and add the paneer. Season with salt and fry until golden on all sides, then remove and set aside.

2. Add the rest of the ghee or oil and the cumin seeds, and once they start to sizzle, add the onion and fry until softened and lightly golden. Add the garlic and ginger and fry for a further 30 seconds.

3. Add the cauliflower, peppers, carrots, courgettes and red chillies and keep adding a little of the stock at a time, reducing it down until the veggies are tender (you may not need to use all the stock).

4. Return the paneer cheese to the pan, with the frozen peas and curry powder, fry for a further couple of minutes until everything is coated in the spices, then squeeze in the lemon juice.

5. Sprinkle with some chopped coriander, if you like.

6. Serve and enjoy!

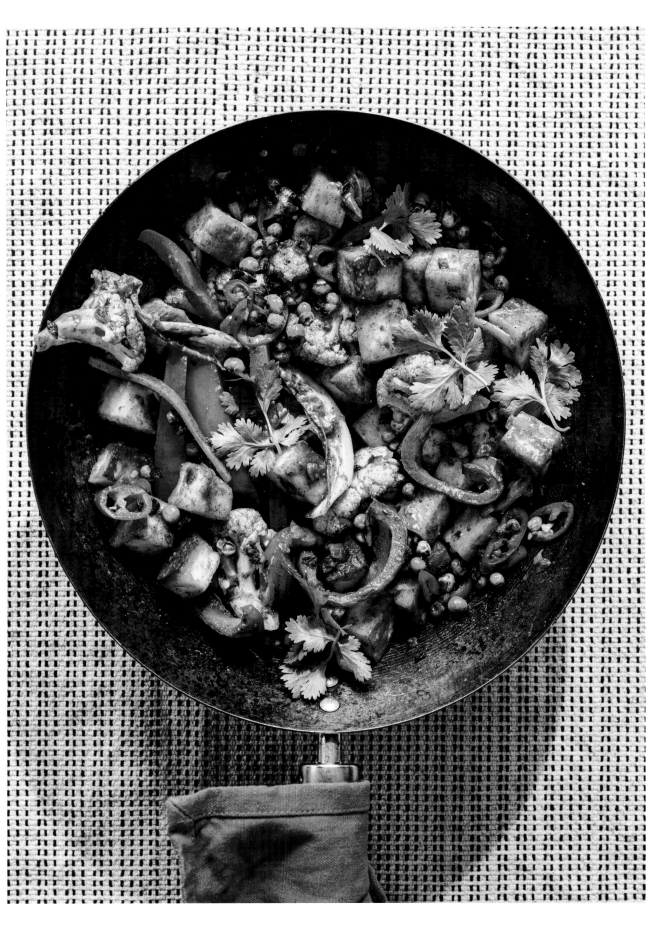

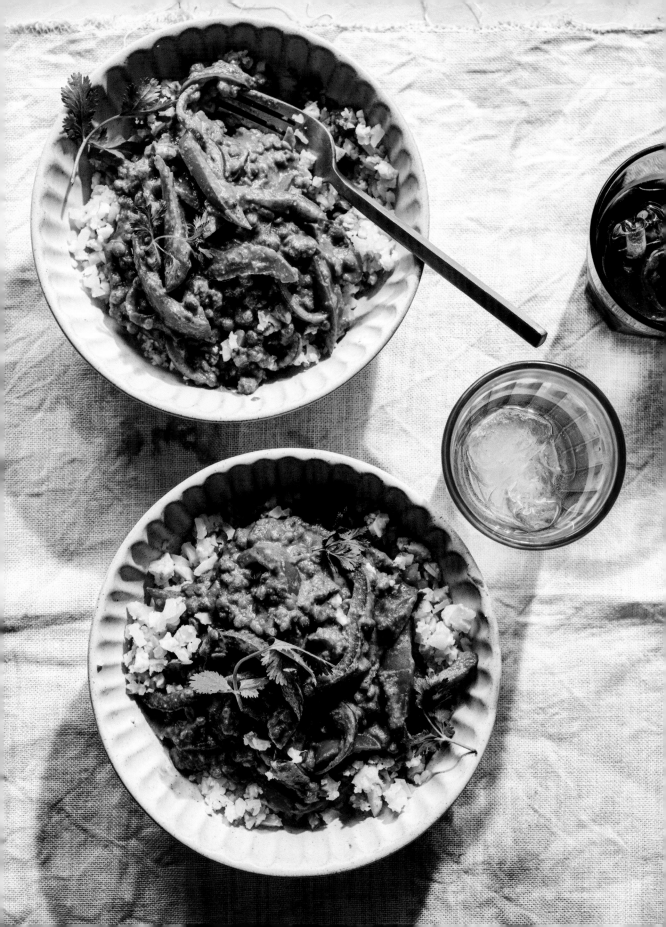

Peanut Lentil Curry

SERVES 4

For the curry paste:
1 small onion, roughly chopped
2 tablespoons tomato purée (paste)
1 thumb-sized piece of fresh ginger, peeled
2 garlic cloves, peeled
2 teaspoons ground cumin
2 teaspoons ground coriander
1 teaspoon chilli powder
½ teaspoon turmeric
pinch of salt
2 tablespoons water

For the curry:
cooking oil spray
1 onion, halved and sliced
1 red pepper, sliced
1 green pepper, sliced
1 x 400g (14oz) tin of green lentils, drained and rinsed
240ml (9fl oz) vegetable stock
3 tablespoons crunchy peanut butter
120ml (4fl oz) light coconut milk
salt and freshly ground black pepper
fresh coriander (cilantro), chopped

Green and brown lentils are a great meat-free substitute for dishes like curries, because they hold their shape. This curry is made with a flavoursome blend of spices and vegetables in a creamy peanut sauce, finished off with a little coconut milk for that extra creamy taste.

1. Put the ingredients for the paste into a mini food processor and whiz to a rough paste.

2. Spray a frying pan with cooking oil.

3. Add the onion and peppers and fry for a couple of minutes to soften, then remove from the pan and set aside.

4. Spray the pan again, then add the paste and cook for a couple of minutes (stirring to ensure it doesn't burn and adding a little water if needed).

5. Add the lentils, stock and peanut butter, bring to the boil, then reduce the heat and simmer for 10 minutes until thickened.

6. Stir in the coconut milk until creamy and return the onion and peppers to the pan.

7. Season as needed with salt and freshly ground black pepper, and sprinkle with chopped coriander.

KCALS
213

FAT
9.9g

SAT FAT
3.5g

CARBS
16.7g

SUGARS
8.1g

FIBRE
9.8g

PROTEIN
9.4g

SALT
0.39g

Gluten-free:
Use gluten-free chilli powder.

Lower-carb side suggestion:
Cauliflower rice (page 239).

Freezing:
To reheat, defrost in the fridge, then warm in a saucepan over a medium heat.

Chickpea, Tomato and Feta Traybake

V

GF

KCALS
234

FAT
9.6g

SAT FAT
3.8g

CARBS
19.0g

SUGARS
8.5g

FIBRE
6.7g

PROTEIN
14.4g

SALT
0.58g

SERVES 4

1 x 400g (14oz) tin of
  chickpeas, drained
  and rinsed
1 teaspoon paprika
1 teaspoon dried oregano
1 teaspoon dried basil
500g (1lb 2oz) grape or
  cherry tomatoes, halved
1 large onion, halved and
  thinly sliced
2 garlic cloves, crushed
1 tablespoon extra virgin
  olive oil
½ tablespoon balsamic
  vinegar (good quality)
salt and freshly ground
  black pepper
150g (5½oz) reduced-fat feta

Side suggestions:
Perfect spooned over crispy
wholemeal (whole wheat)
toast, or served with rice,
pasta or lemon Dijon potato
wedges (page 234).

Lower-carb sides:
Cauliflower rice (page
239), sautéed spiralized
courgettes, or roasted
butternut squash.

If you enjoy a fuss-free traybake, then this chickpea, tomato and feta recipe is for you. The roasted tomatoes with garlic, herbs and chickpeas are polished off with some crumbled salty feta.

1. Preheat the oven to 230°C/210°C fan/450°F/gas 8. Line a baking tray with parchment paper.

2. Toss the chickpeas with the paprika, oregano and basil and put them on the lined baking tray along with the tomatoes, onion and garlic.

3. Drizzle with the extra virgin olive oil and balsamic vinegar and toss everything on the tray to coat.

4. Season with salt and freshly ground black pepper.

5. Bake in the oven for 15 minutes, then remove and crumble the feta over the top.

6. Put back into the oven for an additional 10–15 minutes, until the feta is warmed and the tomatoes are caramelized and softened.

7. Serve and enjoy.

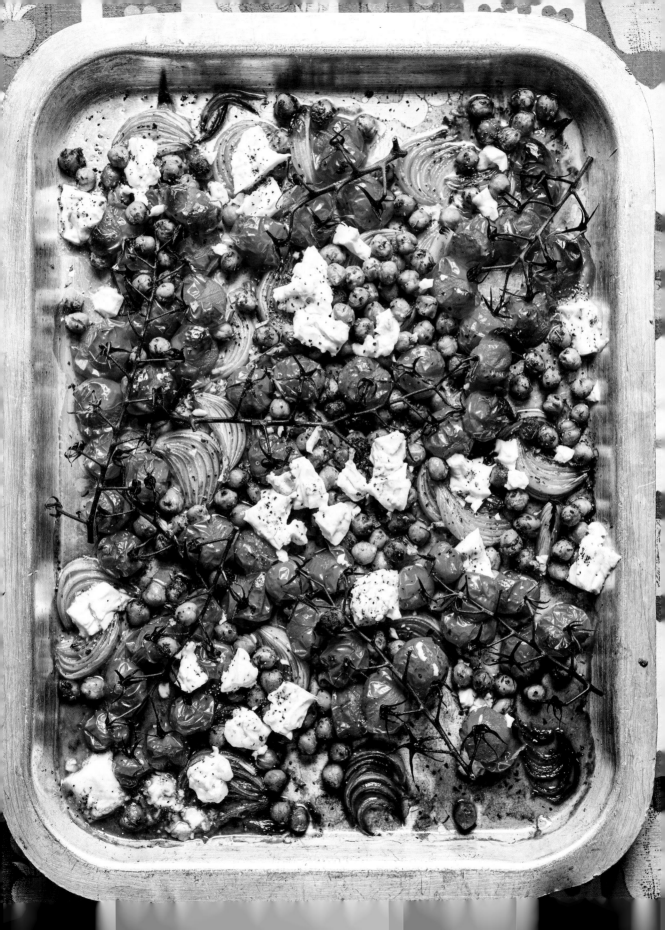

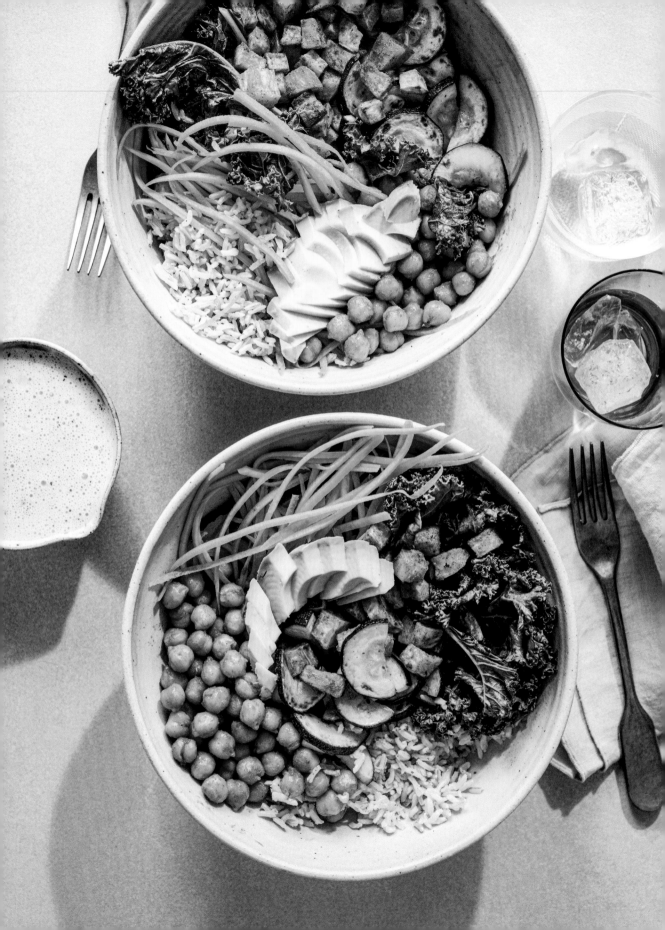

Chickpea Sweet Potato Buddha Bowls

SERVES 2

95g (3½oz) brown rice
720ml (1¼ pints) vegetable
   stock
100g (3½oz) kale, thick
   stems removed
1 small courgette (zucchini),
   approx. 100g (3½oz),
   halved lengthways and
   sliced
olive oil spray
sea salt and freshly ground
   black pepper
1 small carrot, approx. 100g
   (3½oz), thinly cut
70g (2½oz) avocado, mashed

For the sweet potato:
olive oil spray
250g (9oz) sweet potatoes,
   peeled and diced
1 teaspoon paprika
½ teaspoon onion powder
½ teaspoon garlic powder

For the chickpeas:
½ x 400g (14oz) tin of
   chickpeas, drained and
   rinsed
¾ teaspoon paprika
½ teaspoon ground cumin
pinch of salt and freshly
   ground black pepper
juice of ½ lemon
1 tablespoon maple syrup
   or honey

For the dressing:
150g (5½oz) fat-free
   Greek yoghurt
2 tablespoons chopped
   fresh coriander (cilantro)
juice of ½ lime
1 garlic clove, crushed
pinch of sea salt
1 teaspoon maple syrup

When it comes to Buddha bowls, pretty much anything goes – there are no strict rules about what you should or shouldn't add. Typically, though, they are vegetarian and consist of little portions of lots of different things like fresh veggies, whole grains and a good source of protein, all finished off with a complementing dressing or sauce. Buddha bowls are one of my favourite meat-free dishes to make in a hurry when I'm short of time and energy.

1. Preheat the oven to 200°C/180°C fan/400°F/gas 6.

2. Blend the ingredients for the dressing until smooth, and set aside.

3. Line a baking tray with parchment paper, and spray the paper with olive oil. Add the sweet potatoes, paprika, onion powder and garlic powder and toss to coat. Spread out the sweet potatoes on the tray, spray over the top with olive oil, and bake for about 30–35 minutes, until golden and tender.

4. Meanwhile, rinse the rice under cold running water, then put it into a saucepan with the stock. Bring to the boil, then reduce the heat, cover the pan and simmer for about 25–30 minutes, until the rice is cooked. Drain, place back on the hob with the lid on and the heat off, leave for 10 more minutes, then fluff with a fork.

5. Put the kale and courgette into a frying pan (skillet), spray with olive oil and season with salt and freshly ground black pepper. Fry for just a couple of minutes, enough to soften the kale and lightly sauté the courgette.

6. Spray a frying pan (skillet) with olive oil. Add the chickpeas, paprika and cumin, with a pinch of salt and freshly ground black pepper, and fry for a couple of minutes. Squeeze in the lemon juice, add the maple syrup, and continue to heat until the chickpeas are just coated.

7. Once everything is ready, build your bowl: add half the rice, chickpeas, sweet potato, kale, courgette, carrot and avocado to each bowl and drizzle with the lime and coriander dressing.

Dairy-free:
Use a dairy-free yoghurt
for the dressing.

V

GF

KCALS
590

FAT
13.7g

SAT FAT
2.2g

CARBS
83.8g

SUGARS
26.3g

FIBRE
17.1g

PROTEIN
24.4g

SALT
1.11g

Butternut Squash and Ricotta Bake

V

GF

KCALS
317

FAT
15.3g

SAT FAT
8.8g

CARBS
25.6g

SUGARS
16.4g

FIBRE
7.6g

PROTEIN
15.5g

SALT
1.76g

SERVES 4

1 butternut squash, cubed
(approx. 850g/1lb 14oz
once peeled/chopped)
2 teaspoons paprika
250g (9oz) cherry or grape
tomatoes, halved
1 teaspoon fine sea salt
¼ teaspoon freshly ground
black pepper
olive oil spray
1 tablespoon butter
1 large onion, diced
3 garlic cloves, crushed
12 fresh sage leaves,
finely chopped
1 tablespoon tomato purée
(paste)
180g (6oz) ricotta
1 large egg, beaten
30g (1oz) Parmesan or
vegetarian Italian-style hard
cheese, grated
50g (2oz) mozzarella, grated

Side suggestions:
Delicious with rice or pasta.

Lower-carb suggestions:
A simple side salad of mixed
baby leaves.

Freezing:
To reheat after freezing, simply
defrost in the fridge, then
warm through in an oven
preheated to 200°C/180°C
fan/400°F/gas 6, or in a frying
pan over a low heat.

Butternut squash is such a versatile, filling ingredient I like to use often. In this bake it is paired with roasted tomatoes and ricotta cheese, and when you add the sautéed caramelized onions with fresh sage and top with cheese, you have an amazing and super satisfying meal.

1. Preheat the oven to 220°C/200°C fan/425°F/gas 7. Line a large baking tray with parchment paper.

2. Toss the butternut squash with the paprika and place on one side of the lined tray, well spaced out. Put the tomatoes on the other side. Season with the salt and black pepper and spray the top with olive oil.

3. Roast for 30 minutes, until the butternut squash is golden and the tomatoes are soft.

4. In the meantime, melt the butter in a frying pan. Add the onion and fry until golden, add a pinch of salt, the garlic and the sage, and continue to fry until the onion mix is all caramelized (being careful not to burn, and adding a little water and reducing it down if necessary). Set aside.

5. Put the roasted butternut squash into an ovenproof dish. Mix the roasted tomatoes with the tomato purée and spoon this roughly in between the cubes of butternut squash.

6. Mix the ricotta with the onion, sage and garlic mixture and the egg, and spoon this roughly over the butternut squash.

7. Top with the Parmesan and mozzarella and bake until the cheese is golden and melted (approx. 20 minutes).

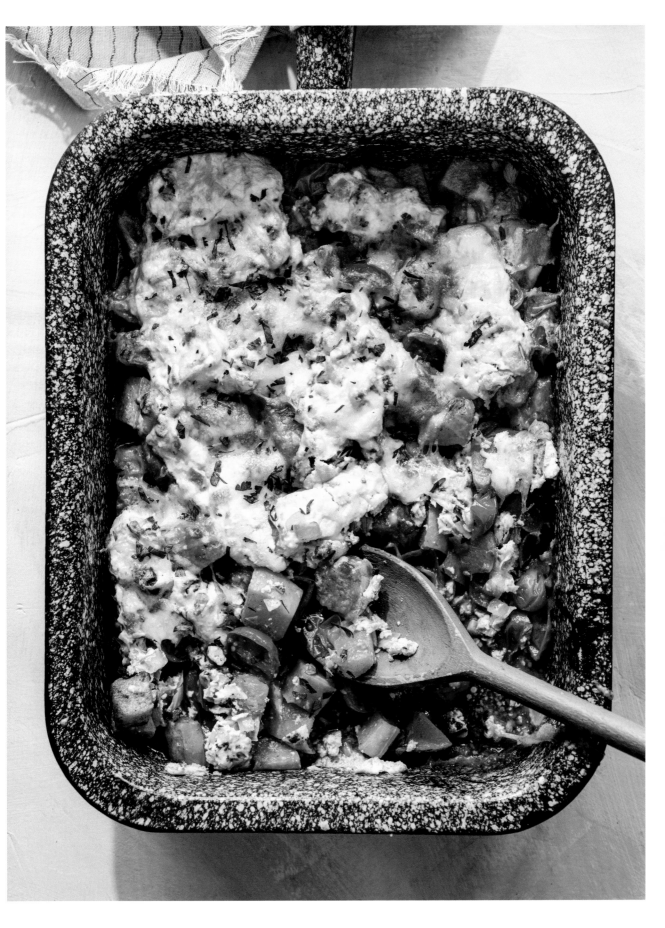

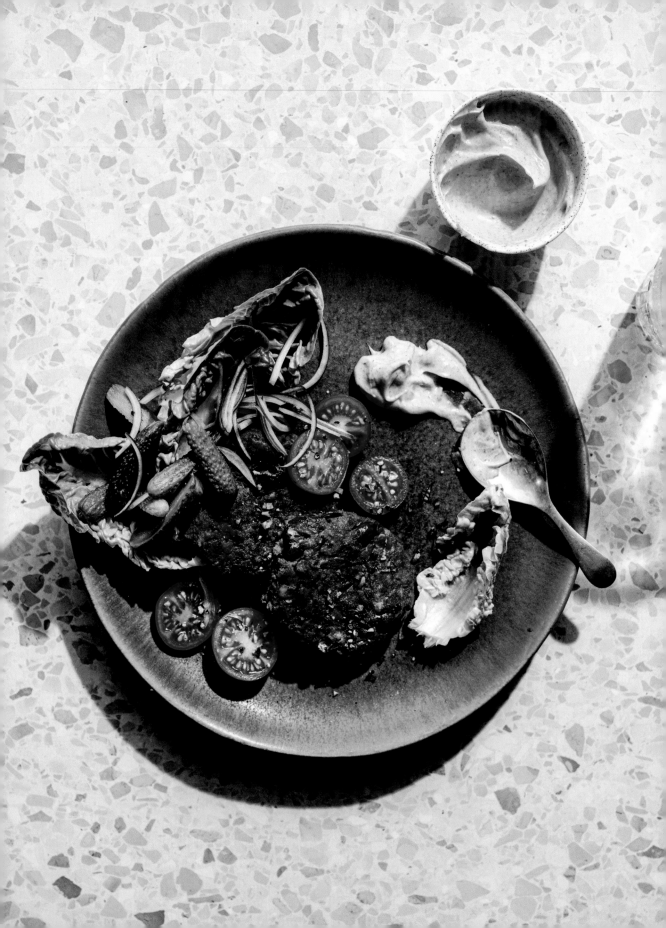

Sweet Potato and Kidney Bean Burgers with Curried Dip

SERVES 4

For the bean burgers:
350g (12½oz) sweet potato
cooking oil spray
75g (3oz) onions, chopped
75g (3oz) carrots, chopped
2 garlic cloves, crushed
1 tablespoon tomato purée
  (paste)
½ tablespoon ground cumin
1 teaspoon paprika
½ teaspoon red chilli flakes
1 teaspoon turmeric
80ml (2½fl oz) water
1 x 400g (14oz) tin of kidney
  beans, drained and rinsed
2 tablespoons chopped
  coriander (cilantro)
salt and freshly ground
  black pepper

For the curried mayo:
6 tablespoons light
  mayonnaise
½ teaspoon lemon juice
¾ teaspoon curry powder
½ teaspoon granulated
  sweetener

Healthy sweet potato and kidney bean burgers are the perfect lunches for work on-the-go or for picnics. These patties combine cooked sweet potato with kidney beans, veggies and spices, and are baked in the oven until lightly golden. Served with the perfect accompaniment – a simple curried dip.

1. Pierce the sweet potato with a knife, place in the microwave and cook for 5 minutes. It should feel soft – remove and set aside.

2. Spray a frying pan with cooking oil, then add the onion and carrot and fry for a couple of minutes to soften.

3. Add the garlic, tomato purée, spices and water, and stir until paste-like and the excess liquid is cooked off. Set aside.

4. Put the kidney beans into a bowl and roughly mash with clean hands or a fork (I find hands much easier). Add the onion and carrot mix.

5. Cut the sweet potato in half and scoop out all the inside. Add the flesh to the bowl with the coriander.

6. Mix together well, until it all binds together, then season with salt and freshly ground black pepper. Form the mixture into 8 burgers.

7. Preheat the oven to 200°C/180°C fan/400°F/gas 6. Line a baking tray with parchment paper and spray with cooking oil.

8. Arrange the burgers on the tray and spray over the top with cooking oil.

9. Bake in the oven for about 12 minutes, then carefully flip and bake for a further 12 minutes.

10. Mix the curried mayo ingredients together in a bowl and serve with the burgers.

Side suggestion:
Serve with a mixed salad. These are also perfect in wholemeal (whole wheat) buns with lettuce, tomato, onion and some of the curried mayo.

Gluten-free:
Use gluten-free curry powder and mayonnaise.

Dairy-free:
Use dairy-free mayonnaise.

Freezing:
Only the burgers are freezer-friendly – freeze after step 6. Defrost in the fridge, then follow steps 7–10.

KCALS
243

FAT
7.4g

SAT FAT
0.7g

CARBS
32.7g

SUGARS
13.7g

FIBRE
10.1g

PROTEIN
6.4g

SALT
0.12g

Taco Veggie Pasta Bake

KCALS
545

FAT
15.2g

SAT FAT
7.1g

CARBS
70.5g

SUGARS
15.2g

FIBRE
14.8g

PROTEIN
24.2g

SALT
1.10g

SERVES 4

olive oil spray
1 onion, finely diced
1 carrot, halved and thinly
    sliced
1 red pepper, diced
1 green pepper, diced
350g (12½ oz) passata
2 tablespoons tomato purée
    (paste)
125g (4½oz) salsa
1 x 400g (14oz) tin of black
    beans, drained and rinsed
1 courgette (zucchini), diced
80g (3oz) frozen sweetcorn
4 tablespoons light
    soured cream
salt and freshly ground
    black pepper
250g (9oz) dried pasta
    (I used fusilli)
100g (3½oz) Cheddar, grated
50g (2oz) black olives, sliced
2 spring onions (scallions),
    sliced

For the taco seasoning:
1½ teaspoons ground cumin
1½ teaspoons paprika
1 teaspoon mild chilli powder
½ teaspoon dried oregano
¼ teaspoon garlic powder
¼ teaspoon onion powder
½ teaspoon cayenne pepper
    (more or less depending on
    your preferred spice level)

The ultimate taco night in a delicious pasta bake. You won't miss the meat in this pasta dish, which is packed with nutritious vegetables and black beans for some added protein in a spicy taco sauce, all rounded off with melted cheese goodness and black olives. Even my veggie-avoiding kids will devour this dish.

1. Mix together the taco seasoning ingredients.

2. Place a frying pan over a medium–high heat and spray with olive oil. Add the onion, carrot and peppers and fry until softened.

3. Add the taco seasoning and stir-fry until coated.

4. Add the passata, tomato purée, salsa, black beans, courgettes and sweetcorn. Then stir in the soured cream until the sauce looks creamy and velvety. Taste the sauce and season with salt and black pepper as needed. Set aside.

5. Add the pasta to a large pan of salted boiling water and cook until al dente. Reserve a third of a cup of the pasta water, then drain off the rest of the liquid.

6. Add the pasta to the sauce and vegetables and toss until coated, adding the reserved pasta water to loosen the sauce if needed.

7. Preheat the oven to 200°C/180°C fan/400°F/gas 6.

8. Put the pasta into an ovenproof dish, top with the grated cheese and scatter over the olives.

9. Bake in the oven for about 30 minutes, until the cheese is all melted and lightly golden.

10. Sprinkle with the chopped spring onions. Enjoy!

Side suggestion:
We serve this with a simple mixed side salad and some additional soured cream.

Gluten-free:
Use gluten-free pasta and chilli powder.

Freezing:
To reheat after freezing, simply defrost in the fridge, then warm through in an oven preheated to 180°C/160°C fan/350°F/gas 4, or in a frying pan over a low heat.

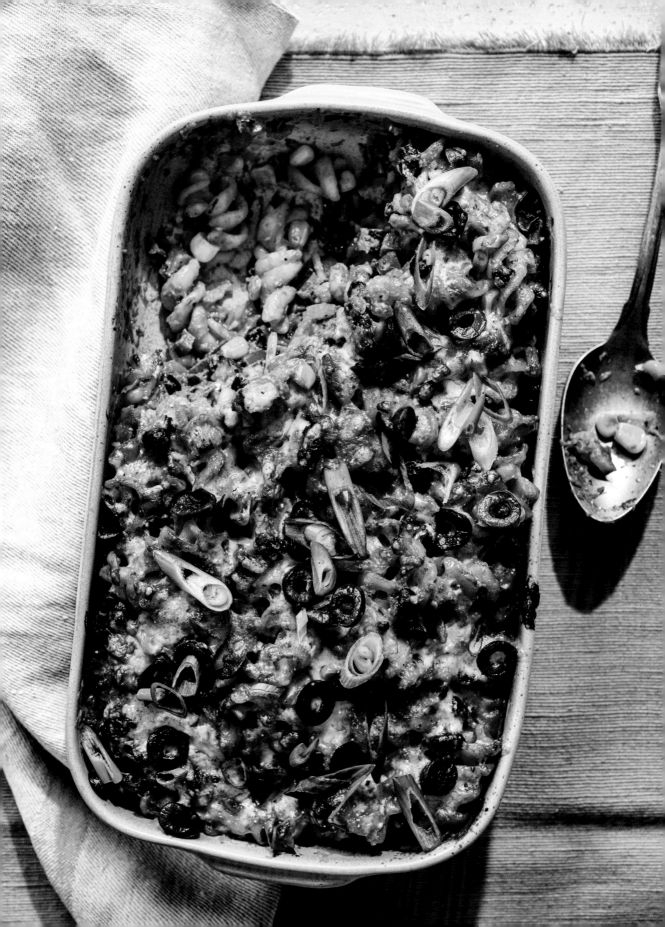

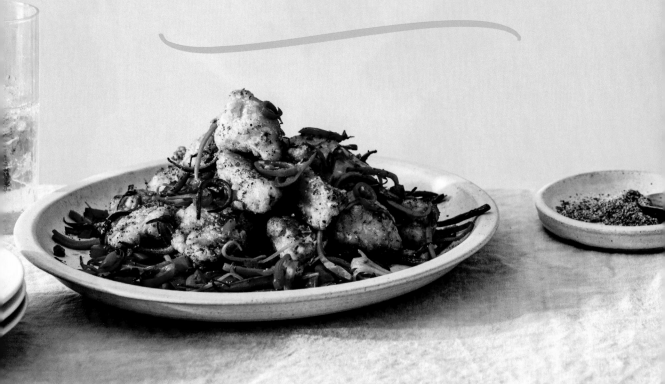

Slimming Eats Favourites

American-style
Oat Pancakes

Ricotta and Spinach
Stuffed Pasta Shells

Leek and Potato Bake

Salt and Pepper
Chicken

Chicken Singapore
Noodles

Chilli Con Carne

Chinese Chicken
Curry

Chicken, Bacon and
Tomato Pasta Bake

Sweet and Sticky Chicken

Balsamic Braised Beef

Best-ever Spaghetti
Carbonara

Yummy Beef and Sweet
Potato Lasagne

Sweet Chilli Beef

Lemon Chilli
Chicken

Pizza Chicken

American-style Oat Pancakes

SERVES 1

40g (1½oz) rolled oats
2 large eggs
4 tablespoons fat-free
    Greek yoghurt
¾ tablespoon granulated
    sweetener
¾ teaspoon baking powder
1 teaspoon vanilla extract
cooking oil spray (I like to
    use coconut for these)
crispy bacon, to serve
    (optional)
fresh fruit, to serve (optional)

Gluten-free:
Use gluten-free
oats and baking powder.

Freezing:
To reheat after freezing,
simply warm through in the
microwave or in a non-stick
frying pan over a medium
heat.

KCALS
384

FAT
14.8g

SAT FAT
3.7g

CARBS
32.1g

SUGARS
3.3g

FIBRE
3.1g

PROTEIN
26.9g

SALT
1.43g

Living in Canada, pancakes are a popular choice for breakfast, so this was one of the first recipes I created on Slimming Eats back in 2009. As a family, our favourite way to enjoy these is with fresh fruit and a drizzle of maple syrup. But for special occasions, it has to be served with a side of crispy smoky bacon. (I'm afraid the bacon is not included in the nutritional count... but so worth it!) Heavenly!

1. Put the oats into a blender and grind to a fine powder.

2. Place in a bowl with the eggs, yoghurt, sweetener, baking powder and vanilla, and mix to combine. Allow to sit for at least 10 minutes.

3. Place a non-stick frying pan over a low heat (make sure you don't have the heat too high) and spray with cooking oil. Add spoonfuls of batter (I use 2 or 3 tablespoons of batter per pancake and I cook 2 pancakes at a time, so that there is enough room in the pan to easily flip them over) and cook until you start to see bubbles appear on the surface, then carefully flip over. A spatula should slide under easily – if it doesn't, the pancakes are not quite done.

4. Repeat with the rest of the mixture.

5. Serve the pancakes with bacon, fruit or toppings of your choice.

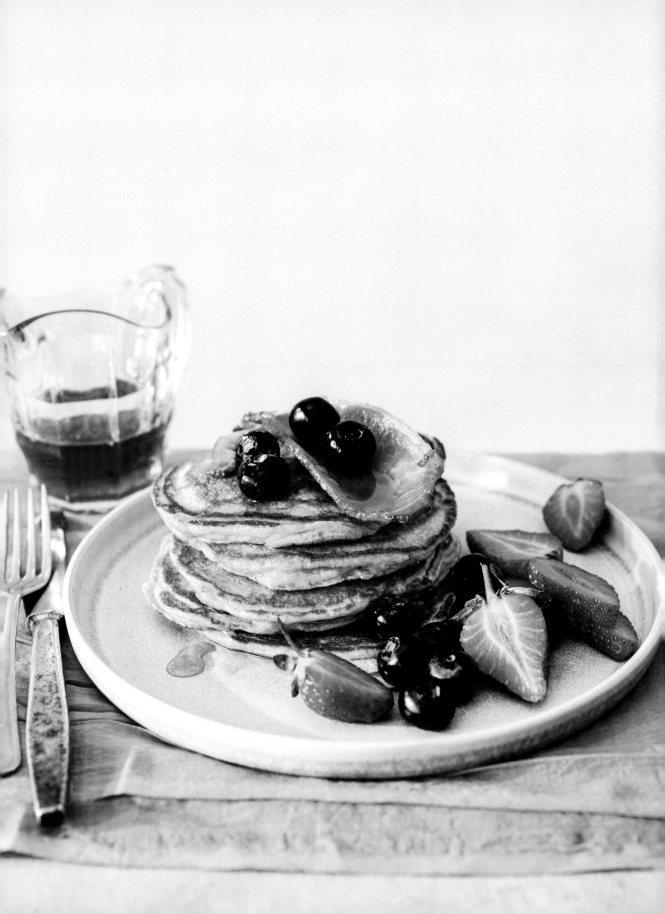

Best-ever Spaghetti Carbonara

KCALS
547

FAT
19.9g

SAT FAT
9.0g

CARBS
52.0g

SUGARS
6.6g

FIBRE
5.0g

PROTEIN
37.5g

SALT
2.49g

SERVES 2

120g (4oz) dried spaghetti
   (you can use gluten-free)
30g (1oz) finely grated
   Parmesan
1 large egg
1 large egg yolk
salt and freshly ground
   black pepper
cooking oil spray
4 slices of lean back bacon
   (fat removed), chopped
1 onion, thinly sliced
2 garlic cloves, crushed
240ml (9fl oz) chicken
   or vegetable stock

To serve:
2 tablespoons chopped
   fresh flat-leaf parsley
30g (1oz) Parmesan, grated

Gluten-free:
Use gluten-free pasta
of choice.

Variations:
You can add some sliced
mushrooms if you like,
when you add the onion
and garlic to the pan.

I guess you could say that readers get excited by my pasta recipes, and this one does not compromise on taste. This is one of my go-to solutions for getting dinner on the table fast. Nothing complicated needed here, just super-accessible ingredients for the most fuss-free, rewarding pasta dish you will ever make.

1. Cook the pasta according to the packet instructions.

2. Drain, but reserve 80ml (2½fl oz) of the cooking liquid.

3. Combine the Parmesan, egg, egg yolk and a little salt and freshly ground black pepper in a small bowl, stirring with a whisk. Gradually add the reserved pasta cooking liquid (this ensures the egg doesn't scramble when you add it to the pasta) to the egg mixture, stirring constantly with a whisk. Set aside.

4. Place a large non-stick frying pan over a medium–high heat and spray with cooking oil. Add the bacon and cook until golden, then remove from the pan and set aside.

5. Add the onion and garlic to the pan and sauté until golden.

6. This is where you will need the stock: if the onions and garlic start to stick, add a little of the stock and continue adding it gradually until the stock is almost gone and the onions have a nice golden colour.

7. Put the pasta and bacon back into the pan, reduce the heat and mix thoroughly.

8. Add the egg mixture, then remove from the heat and toss the pan to evenly coat.

9. Divide equally between 2 plates, season with salt and freshly ground black pepper, and sprinkle with chopped parsley and the rest of the Parmesan before serving.

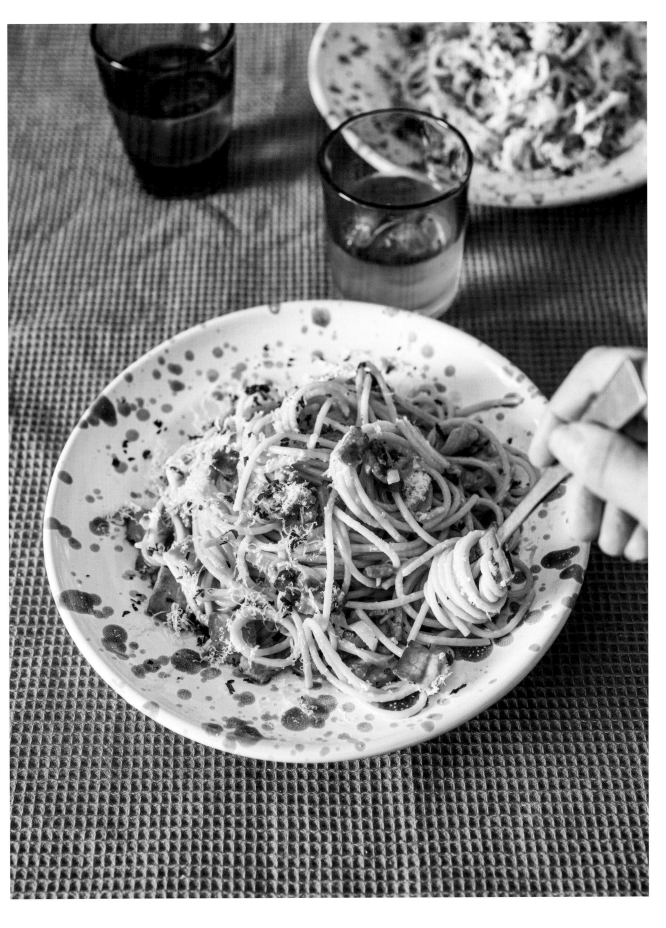

Chicken Singapore Noodles

DF

SERVES 2

cooking oil spray
4 boneless skinless chicken
    thighs (270g/9½oz),
    trimmed of all visible fat
    and sliced into strips
1 tablespoon medium
    curry powder
1 teaspoon turmeric
½ teaspoon garlic powder
½ teaspoon ground ginger
2 teaspoons of sambal oelek
    (chilli paste)
1 small onion, halved and
    sliced
100g (3½oz) mushrooms,
    sliced
1 green pepper, sliced
    into strips
1 red pepper, sliced into strips
1 small carrot, grated into
    long strips
1 tablespoon soy sauce
1 tablespoon rice vinegar
1 tablespoon granulated
    sweetener
100g (3½oz) dried egg
    noodles
2 eggs, beaten
2 spring onions (scallions),
    finely sliced

Gluten-free:
Swap soy sauce and curry
powder for gluten-free
alternatives.

KCALS	**568**
FAT	**16.7g**
SAT FAT	**4.1g**
CARBS	**56.1g**
SUGARS	**14.5g**
FIBRE	**11.6g**
PROTEIN	**42.5g**
SALT	**2.15g**

This delicious curry-flavoured noodle dish will become a regular in your meal plans. Everyone goes wild for these chicken noodles. Traditionally Singapore noodles uses rice noodles, but as a family we love this made with egg noodles. You can vary the dish pretty much every time you make it, by using different proteins like pork or prawns, or even by just doubling up on the veggies.

1. Place a wok over a medium–high heat and spray with cooking oil.

2. Add the chicken, curry powder, turmeric, garlic powder, ginger and sambal oelek and fry until lightly browned. Add a couple of tablespoons of water to make a little sauce around the chicken.

3. Remove from the pan and set aside.

4. Wipe the wok clean, then spray with more cooking oil. Add all the vegetables and fry for about 4 minutes. Add the soy sauce, rice vinegar and sweetener.

5. Cook the noodles according to the package directions.

6. Add the noodles and chicken to the pan of vegetables and mix to combine all the ingredients.

7. Spray a small wok or frying pan over a medium–high heat with cooking oil and add the beaten eggs.

8. Cook until they start to set, then break up with a wooden spoon.

9. Add the egg to the noodles and toss to combine.

10. Serve the Singapore noodles in bowls, topped with the spring onions.

11. Enjoy!

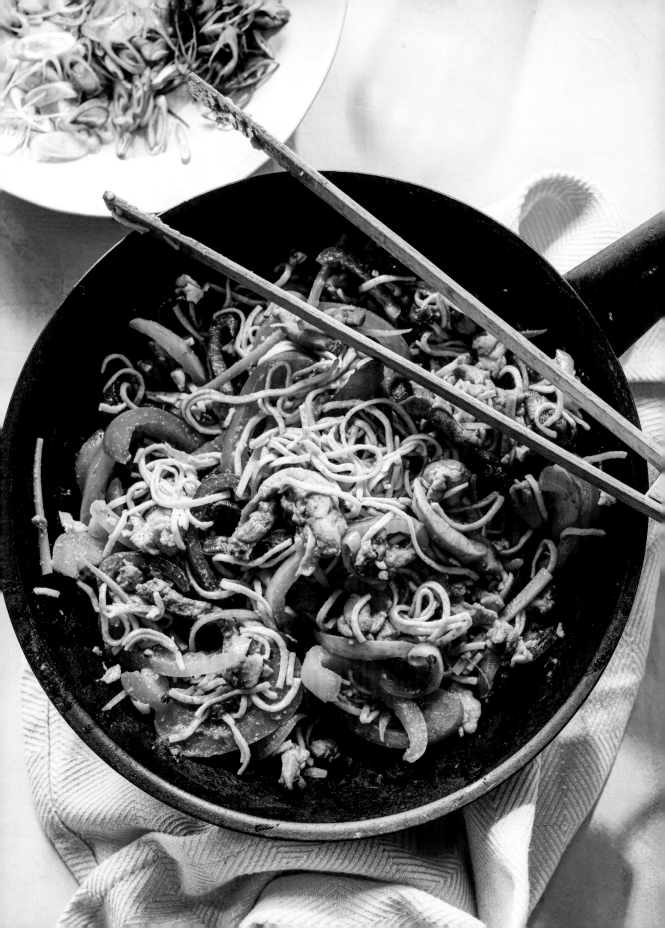

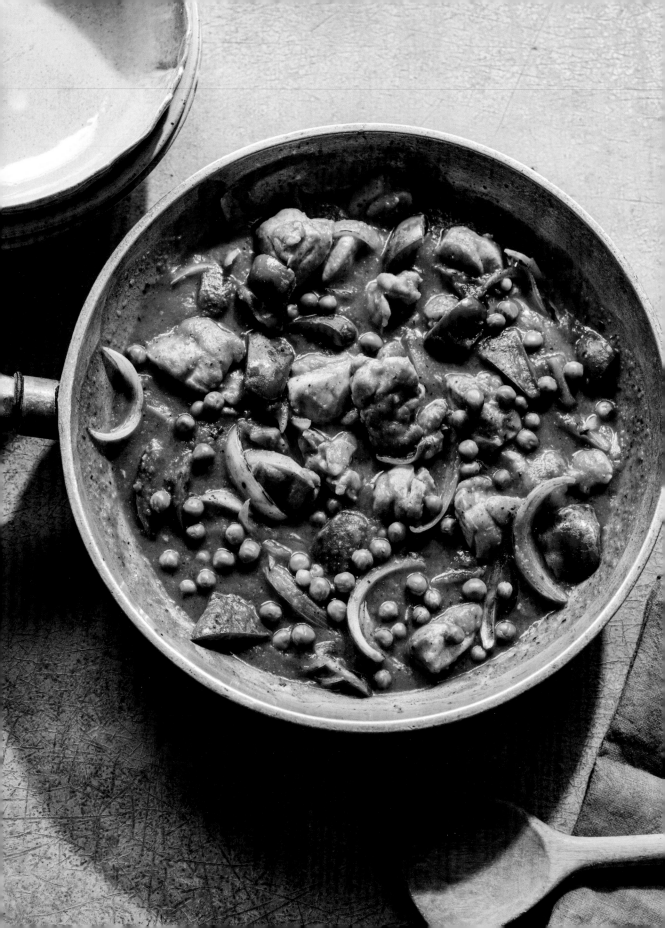

Chinese Chicken Curry

245 Calories

SERVES 4

For the sauce:
cooking oil spray
100g (3½oz) onion, chopped
150g (5½oz) courgette
  (zucchini), chopped
200g (7oz) butternut squash,
  peeled and chopped
1 garlic clove, crushed
1 teaspoon grated fresh ginger
1½ tablespoons curry powder
  (hot or medium, depending
  on how hot you like it)
¼ teaspoon Chinese five-spice
  powder
1 tablespoon tomato purée
  (paste)
1 tablespoon light soy sauce
720ml (1¼ pints) chicken
  stock

For the curry:
450g (1lb) boneless skinless
  chicken breast, diced
1 small onion, chopped
1 green pepper, chopped
80g (3oz) frozen peas

Gluten-free:
Use gluten-free curry
powder.

Lower-carb side:
Serve with the special fried
cauliflower rice (page 239).

Freezing:
To reheat after freezing,
simply defrost in the fridge,
then warm through in the
microwave or in a saucepan
over a medium heat.

This is one of the most popular curry recipes on the blog, and now you can create this takeaway dish from the debut Slimming Eats cookbook. The sauce comes packed with vegetables, so it's another sneaky recipe for fussy eaters. And once you've tried it with chicken, don't be afraid to try it with beef or prawns too.

1. Place a frying pan over a medium–high heat and spray it with cooking oil.

2. Add the onion, courgette and butternut squash and fry for 2–3 minutes, to soften.

3. Add the garlic and ginger and fry for 1 more minute.

4. Add the curry powder, Chinese five-spice, tomato purée and soy sauce, and stir to coat.

5. Pour in the chicken stock, bring to the boil, then cover and simmer for 20 minutes.

6. Transfer to a blender and blend until smooth. Set aside.

7. Spray a frying pan with cooking oil, then add the chicken and fry for about 5 minutes, until lightly browned. Remove from the pan and set aside.

8. Spray the frying pan again, then add the onion and green pepper and fry for 2 minutes.

9. Put the chicken back into the pan, pour in the sauce, stir to coat, and add the peas. Bring to the boil, then cover and simmer for about 5 minutes, until the chicken is cooked through.

10. Serve with your choice of side.

KCALS
245

FAT
5.9g

SAT FAT
1.6g

CARBS
13.2g

SUGARS
8.4g

FIBRE
6.0g

PROTEIN
13.9g

SALT
1.71g

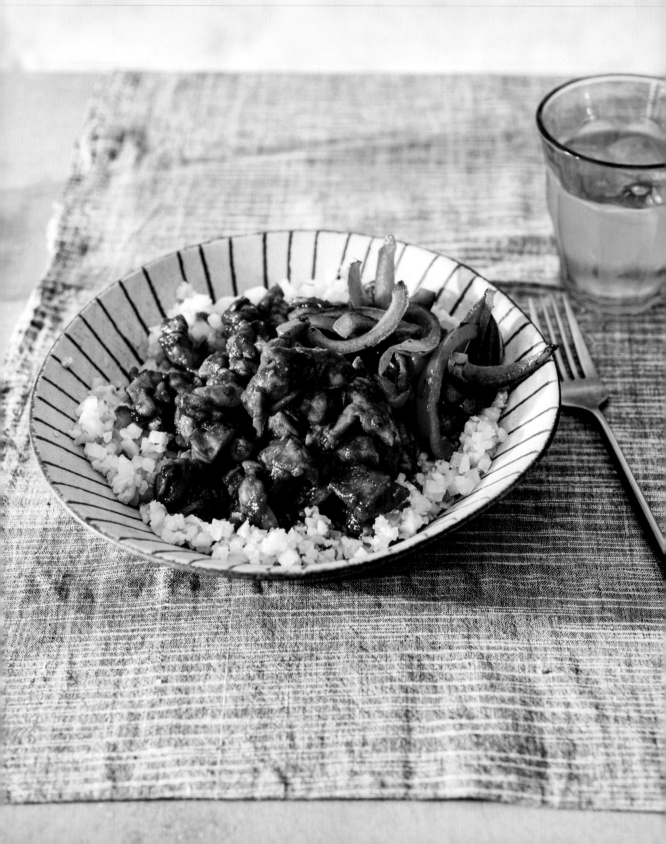

Sweet and Sticky Chicken

SERVES 4

cooking oil spray
750g (1lb 10oz) boneless
    skinless chicken thighs
    (trimmed of all visible fat),
    sliced into strips
1 tablespoon grated
    fresh ginger
½ teaspoon onion powder
½ teaspoon garlic powder
salt and freshly ground
    black pepper

For the sweet and sticky sauce:
120ml (4fl oz) water
4 tablespoons maple syrup
3 tablespoons balsamic
    vinegar
1 tablespoon soy sauce
1 tablespoon tomato purée
    (paste)

Gluten-free: Use gluten-free
soy sauce.

Lower-carb sides: Serve with
cauliflower mash, cauliflower
rice (page 239), or stir-fried
vegetables of your choice.

Freezing:
To reheat after freezing,
simply defrost in the fridge,
then warm through in the
microwave or in a saucepan
over a medium heat.

If you want a easy but tasty chicken recipe – this is it: tender strips of seasoned chicken thighs in a lick-the-spoon sweet and sticky sauce. It's a recipe that's frequently made by Slimming Eats readers. Perfect with many different sides, from rice to potato wedges or even noodles with some stir-fried veggies.

1. For the sauce, combine the water, maple syrup, balsamic vinegar, soy sauce and tomato purée in a jug.

2. Place a frying pan over a high heat and spray with cooking oil.

3. Add the chicken, ginger, onion and garlic powders, and season with salt and freshly ground black pepper.

4. Fry until the chicken is lightly golden on all sides, then remove from the pan and set aside.

5. Add the sauce ingredients to the frying pan and use a wooden spoon to scrape up any bits stuck to the pan – these will add flavour to your sauce.

6. Bubble the sauce on a high heat until it starts to thicken – you will know it is thick enough if you run a wooden spoon through it and the sauce divides.

7. Once the sauce is the right consistency, put the chicken back in and continue to simmer until the chicken is well coated in the sauce and cooked through.

8. Taste and season with salt and freshly ground black pepper.

9. Serve with your choice of sides and enjoy!

292
Calories

KCALS
292

FAT
9.5g

SAT FAT
2.8g

CARBS
16.4g

SUGARS
14.4g

FIBRE
0.3g

PROTEIN
34.8g

SALT
0.82g

Leek and Potato Bake

SERVES 3

GF

V

cooking oil spray
2 large leeks, trimmed,
    sliced and washed
2 garlic cloves, crushed
salt and freshly ground
    black pepper
700g (1lb 9oz) potatoes,
    thinly sliced
60g (2oz) Parmesan or
    vegetarian Italian-style
    hard cheese, grated
120ml (4fl oz) vegetable
    or chicken stock
50g (2oz) mozzarella, grated
chopped fresh parsley

Optional add-ins:
You can add some diced
cooked bacon or ham.

Freezing:
To reheat after freezing,
simply defrost in the fridge,
then warm through in the
microwave or in an oven
preheated to 180°C/160°C
fan/350°F/gas 4.

KCALS
370

FAT
10.5g

SAT FAT
6.4g

CARBS
47.3g

SUGARS
4.5g

FIBRE
8.1g

PROTEIN
17.5g

SALT
0.74g

When we're eating more healthily, we often get stuck in a rut about how to make side dishes more interesting – this leek and potato bake is a popular choice. With inspiration from a potato gratin but without all the calorie-laden cream sauce, it still feels decadent and packed with flavour. Some Slimming Eats readers love this dish so much they will enjoy it as a main course instead of a side. Either way, it's adored by all.

1. Preheat the oven to 200°C/180°C fan/400°F/gas 6.

2. Place a frying pan over a medium–high heat and spray with cooking oil. Add the leeks and garlic and fry until softened. Season with salt and freshly ground black pepper.

3. Put half the leek mixture into an ovenproof dish, then add half the potatoes in a layer. Sprinkle with half the Parmesan.

4. Add the rest of the leeks, then a final layer of potatoes.

5. Pour over the stock.

6. Top with the mozzarella and the rest of the Parmesan and bake in the oven until the top is golden and the potatoes are cooked through (about 40–45 minutes).

7. Sprinkle with chopped fresh parsley and freshly ground black pepper, and serve as a side or as a main.

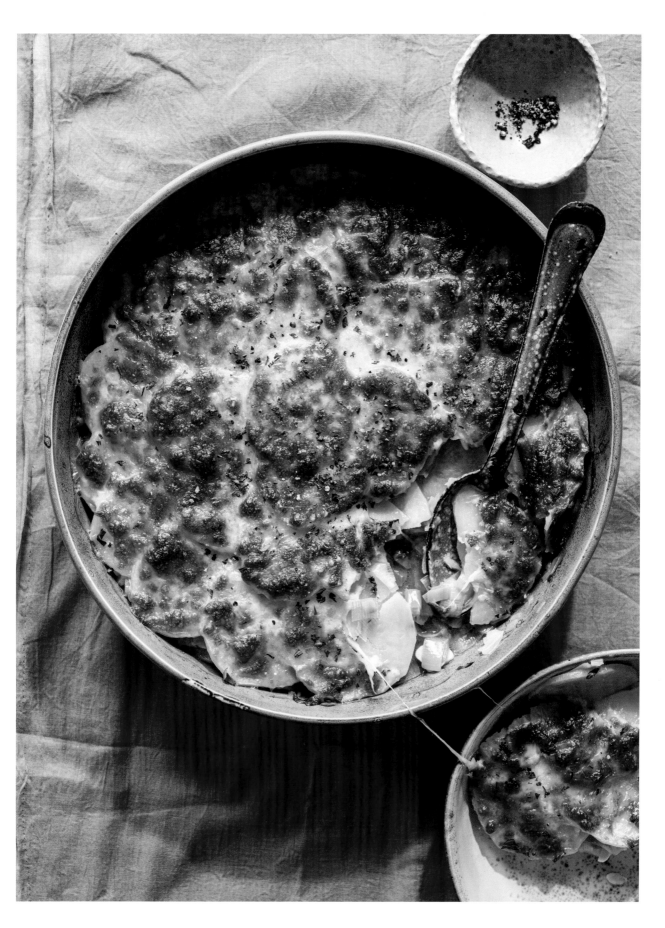

Sweet Chilli Beef

DF

KCALS
225

FAT
10.5g

SAT FAT
4.0g

CARBS
8.4g

SUGARS
5.0g

FIBRE
0.4g

PROTEIN
23.9g

SALT
1.43g

SERVES 4

2 tablespoons sweet
   chilli sauce
2 tablespoons soy sauce
1 tablespoon tomato purée
   (paste)
150ml (5fl oz) water
450g (1lb) beef strips
1 tablespoon cornflour
   (cornstarch) (or tapioca
   or arrowroot)
pinch of salt
2 teaspoons oil of choice
2 spring onions (scallions),
   sliced

Gluten-free:
Use gluten-free soy sauce
and cornflour (cornstarch).

Lower-carb side:
Serve with the special
fried cauliflower rice
(page 239).

It can sometimes be hard to stay motivated when you fancy takeaway food, and that's why I am obsessed with creating lighter versions. This dish is a huge favourite – it combines yummy coated strips of beef in a delicious sweet chilli sauce for your perfect Chinese fakeaway night. Lovely with some stir-fried veggies and homemade egg-fried rice, or, for a healthier side swap, check out the special egg-fried cauliflower rice on page 239.

1. In a bowl, whisk together the sweet chilli sauce, soy sauce, tomato purée and water. Set aside.

2. Pat the beef strips dry with kitchen paper. Put them into a bowl with the cornflour and a pinch of salt and toss to coat.

3. Heat a wok over a medium–high heat. When it's hot, add 1 teaspoon of oil.

4. Add half the beef strips and fry until lightly golden, giving them a light toss occasionally.

5. Remove from the pan and set aside.

6. Add the other teaspoon of oil and repeat with the remaining beef strips. Remove from the pan and add to the other beef strips.

7. Add the sauce ingredients to the pan and heat on medium–high until the sauce just starts to thicken. Lower the heat, return the beef to the pan, and lightly shake the pan to coat the beef in the sauce.

8. Top with the sliced spring onions and serve with your choice of side dish.

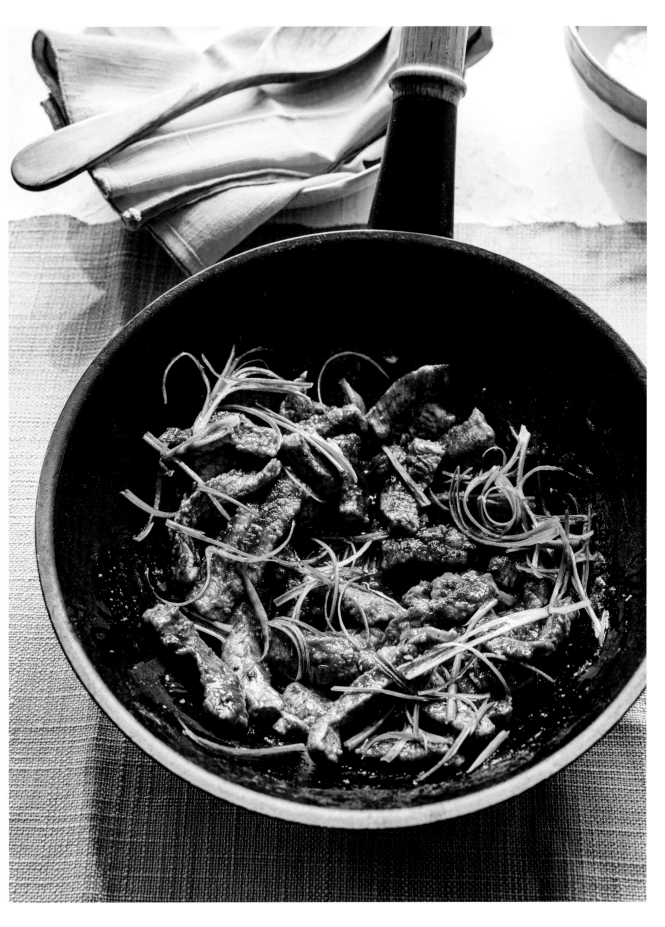

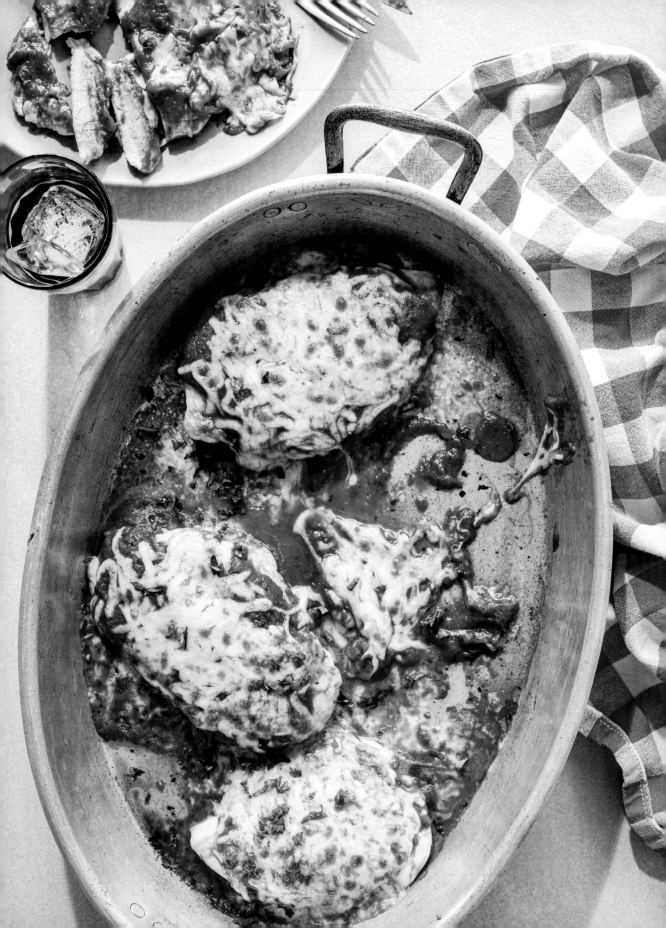

Pizza Chicken

GF

SERVES 4

300g (10½ oz) passata
2 tablespoons tomato purée (paste)
¾ teaspoon onion powder
¾ teaspoon garlic powder
½ teaspoon dried basil
½ teaspoon dried oregano
4 small boneless skinless chicken breasts, flattened
salt and freshly ground black pepper
cooking oil spray
½ tablespoon granulated sweetener (optional, if you prefer a sweeter pizza sauce)
100g (3½oz) mozzarella, grated
chopped fresh parsley

Topping suggestions:

Pepperoni, olives, peppers, mushrooms, onions, ham, pineapple, barbecue sauce instead of pizza sauce, different cheeses (dollops of ricotta are yummy).

Satisfy those pizza cravings with this lower-carb option – the ultimate pizza chicken. Keep it simple with pizza sauce and cheese, or take it to a whole other level with your favourite toppings of choice.

1. Preheat the oven to 220°C/200°C fan/425°F/gas 7.

2. In a bowl combine the passata, tomato purée, onion powder, garlic powder, basil and oregano, and set aside.

3. Season one side of the flattened chicken breasts with salt and freshly ground black pepper.

4. Place a frying pan over a medium–high heat and spray with cooking oil. Once hot, add the flattened chicken breasts (2 at a time, but don't overcrowd the pan if it's not big enough), seasoned side down.

5. Season the top with salt and freshly ground black pepper, and spray with cooking oil.

6. After 2–3 minutes, flip the chicken over – it should be nice and golden – and repeat with the other side.

7. Transfer to an ovenproof dish.

8. Taste the pizza sauce and add the granulated sweetener if using. Pour the sauce over the chicken and scatter over the grated mozzarella.

9. Bake until the cheese has melted and the chicken is cooked through but still tender (approx. 10–12 minutes).

10. If you want the cheese more golden, you can finish the dish under the grill (broiler) for a couple of minutes.

11. Sprinkle with chopped parsley and serve with your choice of sides.

KCALS	**254**
FAT	**9.8g**
SAT FAT	**3.4g**
CARBS	**4.9g**
SUGARS	**4.2g**
FIBRE	**1.3g**
PROTEIN	**35.9g**
SALT	**0.43g**

Ricotta and Spinach Stuffed Pasta Shells

KCALS
327

FAT
12.5g

SAT FAT
6.7g

CARBS
32.4g

SUGARS
6.6g

FIBRE
4.0g

PROTEIN
19.2g

SALT
0.75g

SERVES 4

cooking oil spray
1 small onion, finely chopped
3 garlic cloves, crushed
salt and freshly ground
   black pepper
230g (8oz) spinach,
   chopped
270g (9½oz) ricotta
1 egg
20 jumbo pasta shells
   (approx. 140g/5oz)
30g (1oz) Parmesan or
   vegetarian Italian-style hard
   cheese, grated

For the tomato sauce:
cooking oil spray
1 small onion, chopped
1 garlic clove, crushed
240g (8½ oz) passata
240ml (9fl oz) vegetable
   stock
pinch of mixed herbs

Vegetarian:
Use a vegetarian
Italian-style hard cheese.

Freezing:
To reheat after freezing,
simply defrost in the fridge,
then warm through in the
microwave or in an oven
preheated to 180°C/160°C
fan/350°F/gas 4.

This is one of the top meat-free pasta dishes on Slimming Eats. Everyone falls for the fresh garlicky spinach mixed with ricotta, stuffed into giant pasta shells, and baked in the oven on a bed of tomato sauce until golden.

1. To make the tomato sauce, spray a frying pan over a medium–high heat with cooking oil, add the onion and fry for a couple of minutes until softened.

2. Add the garlic, passata, stock and a pinch of mixed herbs, bring to the boil, then reduce the heat to medium-low and simmer for about 15–20 minutes, until the sauce has reduced down.

3. Allow to cool slightly, then transfer to a blender and blend until smooth. Set aside.

4. Preheat the oven to 180°C/160°C fan/350°F/gas 4.

5. Place a frying pan over a medium–high heat and spray with cooking oil.

6. Add the onion and garlic, season with salt and black pepper, and fry for a few minutes until softened. Reduce the heat and add the spinach, stirring until wilted.

7. Add the ricotta and stir until all combined.

8. Remove from the heat and quickly stir in the egg to prevent it scrambling. Set the mixture aside.

9. Add the jumbo pasta shells to a saucepan of boiling hot water and simmer until al dente (about 8–10 minutes), then drain and allow to cool slightly.

10. Spread the tomato sauce across the bottom of a shallow casserole or other ovenproof dish.

11. Fill the pasta shells with the ricotta and spinach mixture and arrange in the dish on top of the tomato sauce. Sprinkle the Parmesan on top.

12. Place in the oven, covered, and bake for 20 minutes, then remove the cover (or lid) and bake for an another 10 minutes. If you prefer a more golden topping, place under the grill for a couple of minutes before serving.

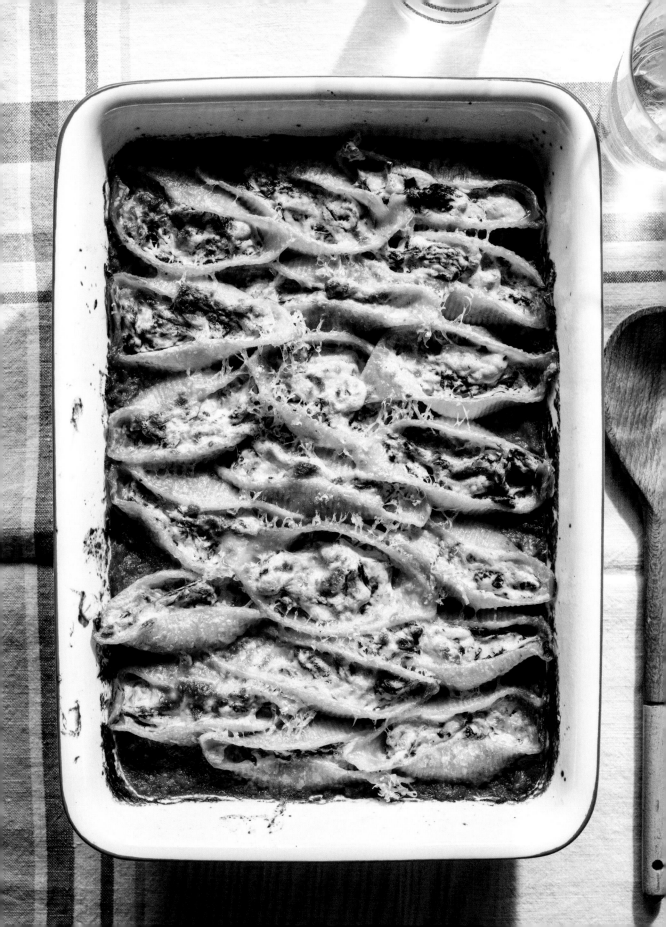

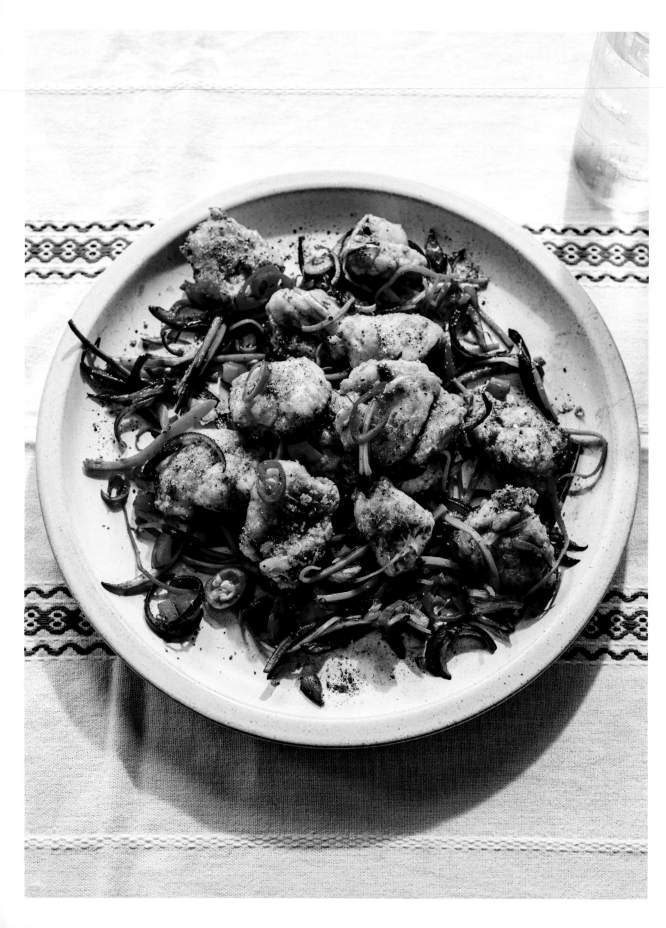

Salt and Pepper Chicken

SERVES 4

For the chicken:
8 boneless skinless chicken
   thighs (approx. 650g/
   1lb 7oz), fat trimmed and
   cut into chunks
salt and freshly ground
   black pepper
1 large egg
4 tablespoons cornflour
   (cornstarch) (or tapioca
   or arrowroot)
cooking oil spray

For the vegetables:
1 red onion, finely diced
3 garlic cloves, crushed
1 red chilli, sliced
½ red pepper
½ green pepper
60ml (2fl oz) chicken stock
1 small carrot, sliced into
   thin matchsticks
1 tablespoon soy sauce
1 tablespoon rice vinegar
2 spring onions, sliced

For the salt and pepper mix:
2 teaspoons fine salt
2 teaspoons freshly ground
   black pepper
2 teaspoons Chinese five-spice
   powder
2 teaspoons granulated
   sweetener

Gluten-free:
Use gluten-free cornflour
(cornstarch) and soy sauce.

Lower-carb side suggestions:
Special fried cauliflower rice
(page 239).

Salt and pepper chicken – tender coated pieces of chicken thigh with the perfect salt and pepper blend. Here's how to create this popular Chinese dish in your own home.

1. Preheat the oven to 200°C/180°C fan/400°F/gas 6 and line a baking tray with parchment paper.

2. Put the chicken into a large bowl and season generously with salt and freshly ground black pepper.

3. Whisk the egg in a separate bowl and pour it over the chicken. Toss well to coat thoroughly, then drain off the excess.

4. Gradually sprinkle in the cornflour, tossing as you do so, until the chicken is well coated.

5. Place the coated chicken on the lined baking tray, spray the top with cooking oil, and bake for 20–30 minutes, until lightly golden.

6. Place a frying pan or wok over a medium–high heat and spray with cooking oil spray. Add the onion and garlic and fry for 1 minute to soften.

7. Add the chilli and the peppers, then gradually add a little stock at a time, continuing to toss the veg as you do so, until it is all absorbed.

8. Add the carrot, soy sauce and rice vinegar, and heat until the liquid evaporates.

9. Mix the salt and pepper seasoning ingredients together in a bowl.

10. When the chicken is done, add it to the pan of vegetables. Sprinkle with some of the salt and pepper mix and toss to coat. Keep doing this gradually with the salt and pepper mix until the chicken is seasoned to your liking. I don't recommend adding the seasoning all at once, as you may want less depending on your taste.

11. Sprinkle with the sliced spring onions and serve with your choice of sides.

DF

KCALS	**320**
FAT	**10.1g**
SAT FAT	**2.9g**
CARBS	**22.3g**
SUGARS	**7.0g**
FIBRE	**3.1g**
PROTEIN	**33.4g**
SALT	**3.39g**

Chilli Con Carne

 DF

 GF

❄

KCALS
264

FAT
5.3g

SAT FAT
2.0g

CARBS
21.4g

SUGARS
12.8g

FIBRE
9.7g

PROTEIN
28.0g

SALT
0.38g

SERVES 6

olive oil spray
500g (1lb 2oz) extra lean
   (5% fat) beef mince
1 onion, finely chopped
3 garlic cloves, crushed
1 carrot, finely chopped
2 teaspoons paprika
2 teaspoons ground cumin
½ teaspoon cayenne pepper
   (optional – omit if you
   don't like it too spicy)
1 teaspoon dried oregano
2 x 400g (14oz) tins of
   chopped tomatoes
150ml (5fl oz) tomato purée
   (paste)
1 red pepper, finely chopped
2 jalapeños, deseeded
   and chopped
1 tablespoon balsamic vinegar
720ml (1¼ pints) beef stock
1 x 400g (14oz) tin of kidney
   beans, drained and rinsed

Low-carb side suggestions:
Cauliflower rice (page 239),
roasted butternut squash or
enjoy just as it is in a bowl
with a few of your favourite
toppings.

Freezing:
To reheat after freezing,
simply defrost in the fridge,
then warm through in the
microwave or in a saucepan
over a medium heat.

Who doesn't like tucking into a bowl of chilli con carne? It's an all-time classic family-friendly recipe that is regularly featured on meal plans and is one of the most loved recipes from Slimming Eats. Minced beef and kidney beans in a gorgeous blend of spices with a rich sauce – it's pure comfort in a bowl. Whenever I make this, it's served in the middle of the table with various toppings such as Cheddar, soured cream, avocado, spring onions (scallions), salsa, rice, salad, so we can all dig in ourselves and build our own chilli con carne bowl.

1. Spray a large casserole dish over a medium–high heat with some olive oil.

2. Add the mince, onion and garlic and fry until browned.

3. Add the carrot and fry for a further few minutes.

4. Add the spices, oregano, chopped tomatoes, tomato purée, red pepper, jalapeños, balsamic vinegar and stock, and bring to the boil.

5. Reduce the heat to a simmer, add the kidney beans, then cover and cook for about 45 minutes, until the sauce has reduced and thickened.

6. Enjoy!

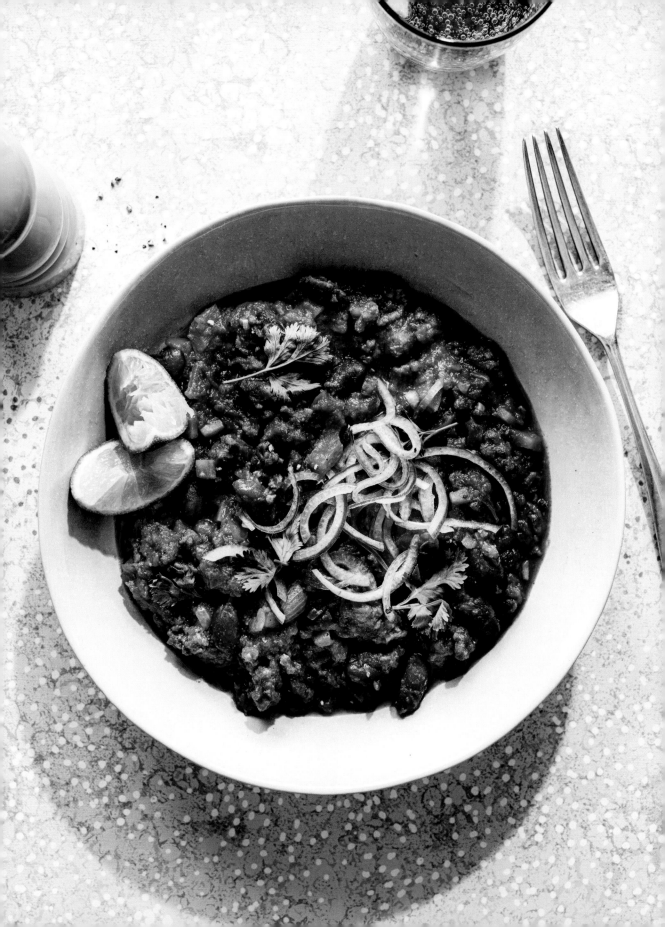

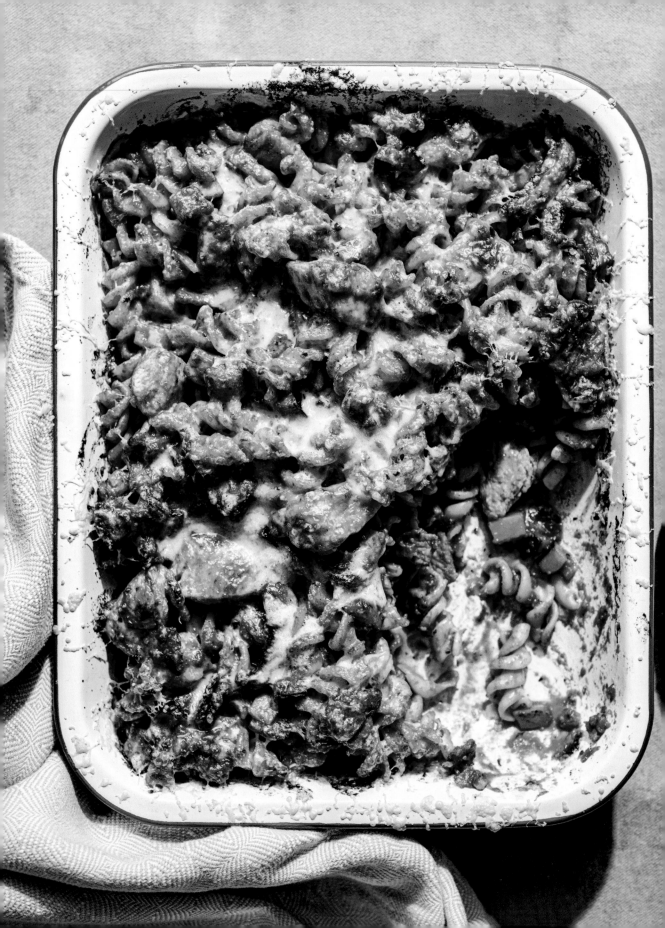

Chicken, Bacon and Tomato Pasta Bake

SERVES 4

200g (7oz) dried penne or fusilli pasta
cooking oil spray
2 skinless chicken breasts (fat trimmed), cut into bite-sized pieces (approx. 350g/12½oz)
1 onion, finely chopped
4 garlic cloves, finely chopped
3 slices of lean bacon (fat removed), finely chopped
1 courgette (zucchini), finely chopped
1 carrot, finely chopped
7 button mushrooms, sliced
handful of cherry or grape tomatoes, halved
480g (1lb 1oz) passata
240ml (9fl oz) chicken stock
splash of balsamic vinegar
splash of Tabasco sauce
2 tablespoons tomato purée (paste)
2 teaspoons dried oregano
salt and freshly ground black pepper
120g (4oz) Cheddar (or you can use mozzarella), grated

Gluten-free
Use gluten-free pasta.

Freezing
To reheat after freezing, simply defrost in the fridge, then warm through in the microwave or in an oven preheated to 180°C/160°C fan/350°F/gas 4.

Winner winner chicken dinner! This combo of chicken and bacon is packed with veggies in the pasta sauce and topped with melted cheese. What's not to like? When my kids were going through a vegetable aversion (most do) I would cook the sauce separately and blend it all up until smooth – it's a great way to sneak vegetables into a meal.

1. Preheat the oven to 200°C/180°C fan/400°F/gas 6.

2. Add the pasta to a saucepan of boiling hot water and cook according to packet instructions until al dente, then drain and rinse with cold water to prevent it cooking further.

3. Place a frying pan on a medium heat and spray with cooking oil. Add the chicken and cook until golden brown, then remove from the pan and set aside.

4. Add the onion, garlic and bacon and cook for 2 minutes.

5. Add the courgette, carrot, mushrooms and tomatoes and cook for a further 5 minutes.

6. Add the passata, stock, balsamic vinegar, Tabasco, tomato purée and oregano and bring to the boil, then reduce the heat and simmer, covered, for about 20 minutes.

7. Transfer the mixture to a casserole dish, along with the pasta and chicken. Season with salt and freshly ground black pepper, top with the Cheddar, and bake in the oven for about 30 minutes, until the cheese on top is melted and golden, then serve.

518 Calories

KCALS
518

FAT
16.2g

SAT FAT
7.2g

CARBS
44.6g

SUGARS
11.9g

FIBRE
7.2g

PROTEIN
44.7g

SALT
2.11g

Balsamic Braised Beef

DF

GF

KCALS
372

FAT
9.0g

SAT FAT
3.1g

CARBS
26.4g

SUGARS
21.4g

FIBRE
5.0g

PROTEIN
43.8g

SALT
0.31g

SERVES 4

cooking oil spray
800g (1lb 12oz) lean stewing beef (fat removed), cubed
1 onion, quartered and sliced
2 garlic cloves, crushed
3 carrots, cut into batons
1 red pepper, chopped
60ml (2fl oz) good-quality balsamic vinegar
2 tablespoons brown sugar
240ml (9fl oz) beef stock
3 tablespoons tomato purée (paste)
pinch of dried thyme
pinch of dried parsley
salt and freshly ground black pepper
1 tablespoon cornflour (cornstarch) (or tapioca or arrowroot)
fresh parsley, chopped

Lower-carb suggestion:
Serve with cauliflower rice (page 239), celeriac (celery root) mash or your favourite steamed/roasted vegetables (my favourites are cauliflower, broccoli and butternut squash).

Freezing: To reheat after freezing, simply defrost in the fridge, then warm through in the microwave or in a saucepan over a medium heat.

This comforting, filling bowl of balsamic braised beef is pure comfort food and a Slimming Eats classic. Tender chunks of beef in a tangy rich tomato sauce, it's made even better with a variety of different sides, such as the rustic kale and leek potato mash on page 255.

1. Place a large casserole dish over a medium heat and spray with cooking oil.

2. Add the beef and brown lightly, then remove from the casserole and set aside.

3. Add the onion, garlic and carrots and continue to fry for a few minutes, adding a little water to deglaze the pan if they stick.

4. Add the rest of the ingredients apart from the cornflour and parsley, bring to the boil, then cover and simmer for about 1½ hours.

5. Mix the cornflour with a little water to make a slurry and stir into the stew until thickened.

6. Sprinkle with chopped parsley and serve with your choice of sides.

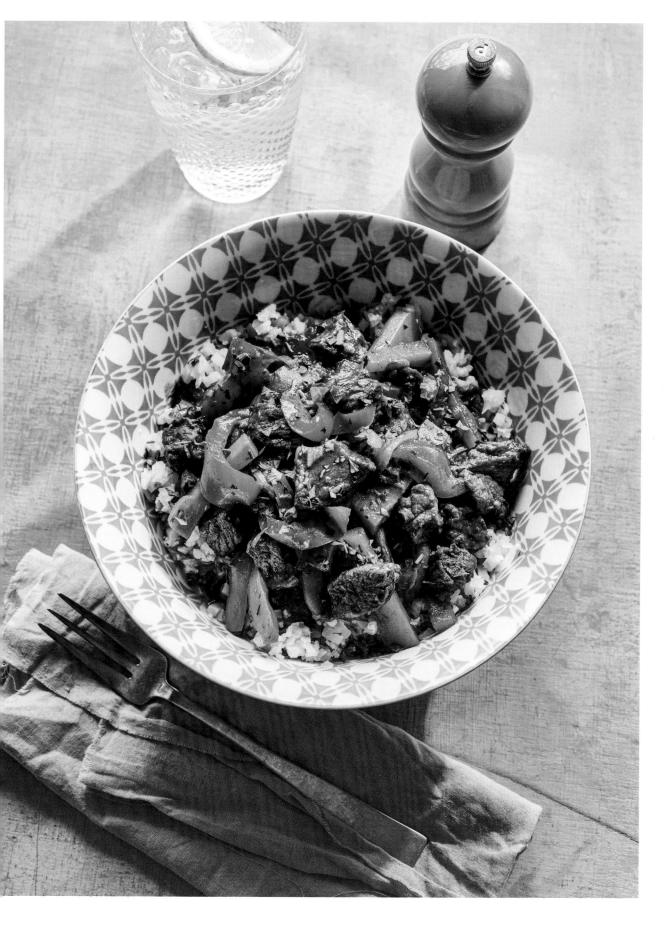

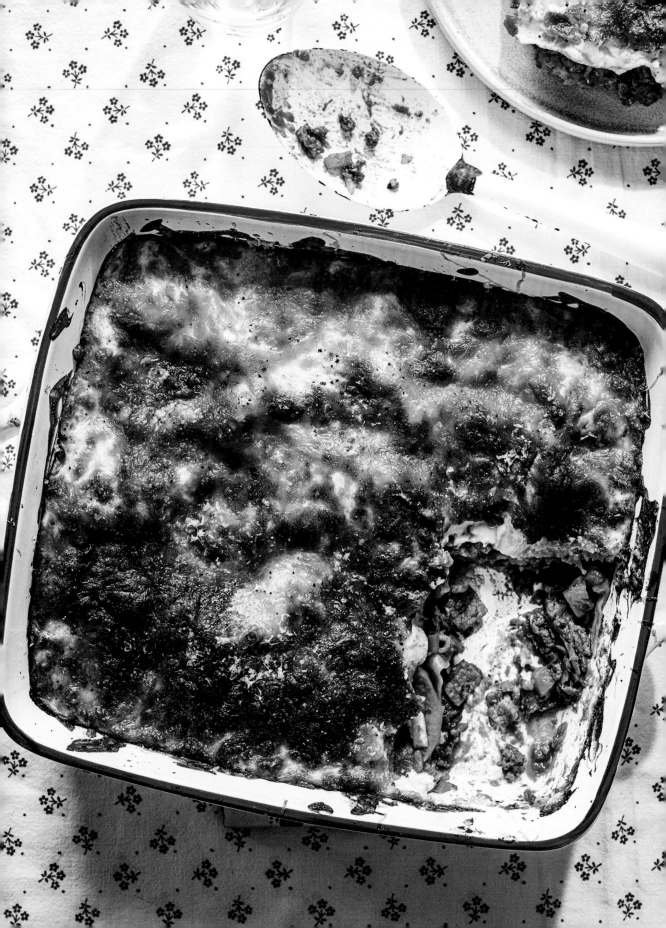

Yummy Beef and Sweet Potato Lasagne

578 Calories

SERVES 4

cooking oil spray
2 slices of lean back bacon
(fat removed), chopped
pinch of ground cinnamon
1 large sweet onion, chopped
4 garlic cloves, crushed
1 carrot, chopped
pinch of fresh chopped herbs
(thyme, oregano, sage,
rosemary)
400g (14oz) extra lean
(5% fat) beef mince
4 mushrooms, chopped
600g (1lb 5oz) tinned
chopped tomatoes or
passata
1 tablespoon tomato purée
(paste)
240ml (9fl oz) beef or
vegetable stock
1 tablespoon balsamic or
red wine vinegar
600g (1lb 5oz) sweet
potatoes, peeled and
sliced into rounds
2 teaspoons paprika
pinch of chilli powder
6 oven-ready lasagne sheets
100g (3½oz) mozzarella,
grated or torn into pieces
15g (½oz) Parmesan, grated

For the cheese sauce:
300ml (10fl oz) 1% milk
4 teaspoons cornflour
(cornstarch)
15g (½oz) Parmesan, grated
salt and freshly ground
black pepper

Freezing:
To reheat, defrost in the
fridge, then warm through in
an oven preheated to 180°C/
160°C fan/350°F/gas 4.

Most people may be put off making lasagne when trying to eat more healthily, but this one will totally change your mind. It's lighter in calories but still has that luxurious lasagne flavour you expect – a rich beef sauce between layers of pasta and sweet potato, rounded off with a healthier béchamel white sauce and melted cheese.

1. Preheat the oven to 200°C/180°C fan/400°F/gas 6.

2. Spray a frying pan with some cooking oil and cook the bacon with a pinch of cinnamon until golden.

3. Add the onion, garlic, carrot and herbs and fry for a further few minutes.

4. Add the beef mince and cook until browned.

5. Add the mushrooms, tomatoes, tomato purée, stock and balsamic vinegar. Bring to the boil, then reduce the heat to low, cover and simmer for about 30 minutes.

6. Put the sweet potato slices on a baking tray and sprinkle with the paprika and chilli powder. Spray the top with cooking oil and bake in the oven until tender (approx. 30 minutes).

7. When the sweet potatoes are almost done, make the cheese sauce.

8. Put the milk and cornflour into a small saucepan over a medium-high heat, constantly stirring until it comes to the boil and thickens. Add the Parmesan and continue to stir until the cheese is melted into the sauce, then season with salt and black pepper.

9. Using a square lasagne dish, make a layer of half the meat mixture. Cover with 3 lasagne sheets, then the sweet potato slices. Repeat with another layer of meat sauce, then another 3 lasagne sheets.

10. Pour the cheese sauce over the top and sprinkle with the mozzarella and Parmesan.

11. Bake for about 30 minutes, until the cheese has melted and is golden. Serve with your choice of sides.

KCALS	**578**
FAT	**14.7g**
SAT FAT	**8.2g**
CARBS	**62.6g**
SUGARS	**28.3g**
FIBRE	**9.4g**
PROTEIN	**43.9g**
SALT	**1.52g**

231 Calories

Lemon Chilli Chicken

DF

KCALS
231

FAT
10.3g

SAT FAT
2.9g

CARBS
5.3g

SUGARS
3.6g

FIBRE
2.9g

PROTEIN
28.0g

SALT
0.93g

SERVES 3

6 skinless chicken thighs
(either bone-in or boneless)
(fat trimmed)
3 garlic cloves, crushed
1 teaspoon grated fresh
ginger
1 onion, finely sliced
1½ teaspoons ground cumin
1 teaspoon mild chilli powder
1 teaspoon ground coriander
½ teaspoon turmeric
cooking oil spray (I used
avocado)
360 ml (12fl oz) chicken
stock
zest and juice of ½ a lemon
salt and freshly ground
black pepper
lemon slices and chopped
fresh coriander (cilantro),
to garnish

Gluten-free:
Use gluten-free
chilli powder.

Freezing:
To reheat after freezing,
simply defrost in the fridge,
then warm through in the
microwave or in a saucepan
over a medium heat.

When you want a healthy meal on the table that doesn't take hours to prepare and cook, this is a great choice. Tender pieces of chicken in a citrusy, spicy lemon sauce, it's one of my go-to chicken recipes because it's pure simplicity. And if you want to take this meal to a whole other level of flavour, a side dish to complement this would be the Indian roasted cauliflower pilau rice on page 256.

1. Put the chicken thighs, garlic, ginger, onion and spices into a large dish and mix well to evenly coat.

2. Place a frying pan over a medium–high heat and spray with cooking oil.

3. Add the chicken and fry until lightly golden.

4. Add the chicken stock, lemon zest and lemon juice to the pan. Increase the heat until it starts bubbling, then reduce to medium so it gently simmers until the sauce reduces down and thickens (don't add a lid) – about 20 minutes. Add a little water if needed to loosen the sauce if it becomes too dry.

5. Season with salt and freshly ground black pepper.

6. Top with fresh lemon slices and chopped coriander, and serve with your choice of sides.

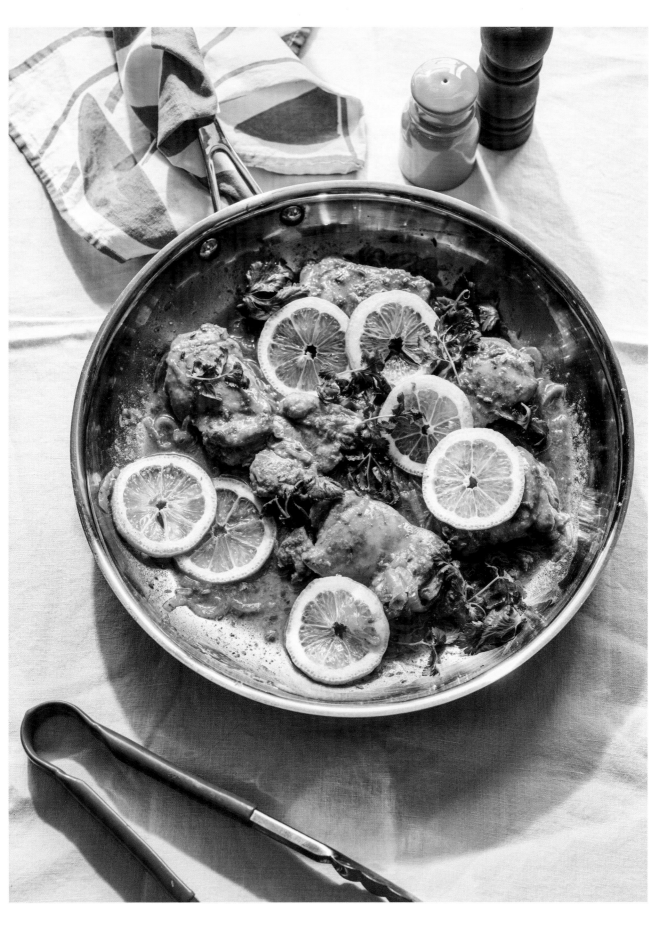

Sides

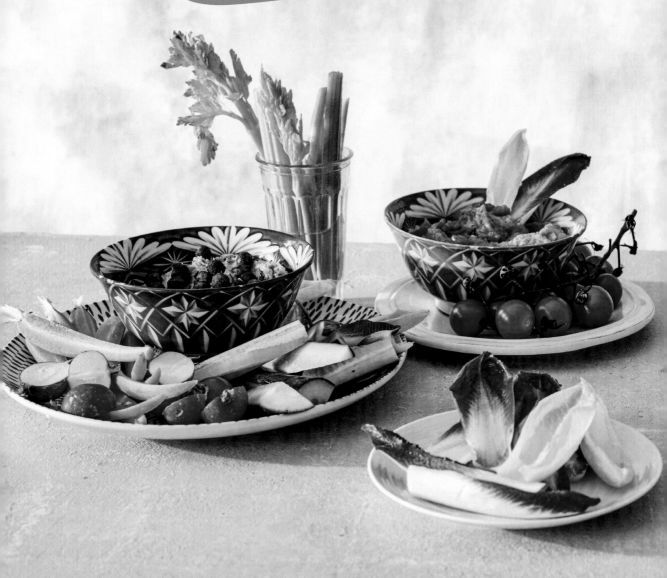

Lemon Dijon
Potato Wedges

Garlic Sauce

Hummus 3 Ways

Cauliflower Rice
3 Ways

Cauliflower Cheese

Potato Latkes

Sumac-roasted
Butternut Squash with
Tahini Dressing

Jalapeño Poppers

Smashed Cheddar
Broccoli with
Ranch Dip

Creamed Spinach

Rustic Kale and Leek
Potato Mash

Indian Roasted
Cauliflower
Pilau Rice

Lemon Dijon Potato Wedges

194 Calories

KCALS: **194**

FAT: **3.6g**

SAT FAT: **0.6g**

CARBS: **33.8g**

SUGARS: **2.7g**

FIBRE: **4.5g**

PROTEIN: **4.5g**

SALT: **1.68g**

SERVES 4

800g (1lb 12oz) waxy
   potatoes
1 tablespoon olive oil
juice and zest of 1 lemon
1 tablespoon Dijon mustard
1 teaspoon dried oregano
1 teaspoon salt
1 teaspoon garlic powder
1 teaspoon onion powder

Optional:
Serve with a little crumbled
feta, grated Cheddar or
vegetarian Italian-style hard
cheese.

These golden lemon Dijon potato wedges are the fail-safe side dish to accompany a variety of main courses. They're also pretty amazing just as they are, straight from the oven, or, if you want a more indulgent side, sprinkle over some crumbled feta, grated Cheddar or vegetarian Italian-style hard cheese.

1. Put the potatoes into a large bowl, cover them with cold water, and leave for about 40 minutes. Drain, rinse thoroughly, pat completely dry, then slice into wedges.

2. Preheat the oven to 220°C/200°C fan/425°F/gas 7. Line a large baking tray with parchment paper.

3. Put the potato wedges on the lined tray.

4. Whisk together the olive oil, lemon juice and zest, mustard, oregano, salt, garlic powder and onion powder.

5. Add to the tray and toss to coat the potatoes, then spread them out in an even layer.

6. Bake for 40 minutes, until golden (remove at the halfway mark, flip them over, and spray with olive oil).

7. Season with more salt as needed.

Garlic Sauce

42 Calories

KCALS: **42**

FAT: **2.1g**

SAT FAT: **0.2g**

CARBS: **2.1g**

SUGARS: **1.7g**

FIBRE: **0.1g**

PROTEIN: **3.6g**

SALT: **0.16g**

SERVES 4

2 tablespoons light
   mayonnaise
3 tablespoons fat-free
   Greek yoghurt
1 garlic clove, minced
a little lemon juice
pinch of salt
½ tablespoon chopped
   fresh parsley

I originally created this sauce to go with the ćevapi on page 136, but it works well as a dipping sauce, or you can drizzle it over your favourite dishes for an extra garlicky kick.

1. Mix together the ingredients for the garlic sauce in a bowl until combined.

2. Serve immediately or store in the fridge until needed. In an airtight container it will last up to 3 days.

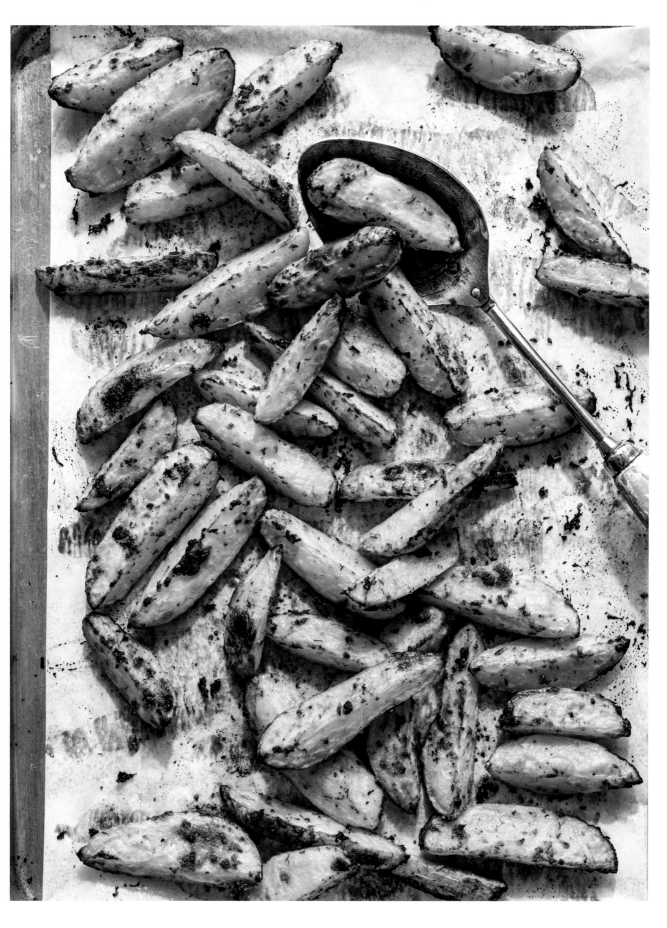

Hummus 3 Ways

Hummus is a staple in our house. There are so many variations and it is super-easy to make at home, perfect for snacks and parties. Here are three of our favourites. Serve them with veggies, crudités, crackers or wholemeal (whole wheat) pita bread.

75
Calories

KCALS: **75**

FAT: **3.3g**

SAT FAT: **0.4g**

CARBS: **6.5g**

SUGARS: **0.3g**

FIBRE: **2.6g**

PROTEIN: **3.6g**

SALT: **0.09g**

Original Hummus

SERVES 6

1 x 400g (14oz) tin of
   chickpeas, drained,
   liquid reserved
1 garlic clove, peeled
1 tablespoon tahini
¾ teaspoon ground cumin
juice of ½ a lemon
pinch of sea salt
pinch of paprika
pinch of sumac
olive oil spray
1 teaspoon extra virgin olive oil
finely chopped fresh parsley

1. Set aside 2 tablespoons of the drained chickpeas.

2. Put the rest of the chickpeas into a food processor with the garlic, tahini, cumin and lemon juice, and pulse. Keep adding a little of the reserved chickpea liquid until it's the consistency you like.

3. Taste and season with a pinch of sea salt.

4. Put the reserved chickpeas into a frying pan with the paprika and sumac and spray with olive oil. Fry until lightly golden, then remove from the heat.

5. Put the hummus into a bowl. Smooth over the top with a spatula, making some ridges in the hummus, top with the reserved chickpeas, then drizzle the olive oil over the top and sprinkle with finely chopped parsley.

116
Calories

KCALS: **116**

FAT: **3.8g**

SAT FAT: **0.5g**

CARBS: **13.4g**

SUGARS: **5.7g**

FIBRE: **4.8g**

PROTEIN: **4.6g**

SALT: **0.28g**

Caramelized Onion Hummus

SERVES 6

olive oil spray
2 large red onions, sliced
240ml (9fl oz) vegetable
   stock
1 tablespoon balsamic
   vinegar
1 x 400g (14oz) tin
   of chickpeas, drained,
   liquid reserved
1 garlic clove
½ teaspoon ground cumin
juice of ½ a lemon
1 tablespoon tahini
pinch of salt
1 teaspoon extra virgin
   olive oil

1. Spray a saucepan with olive oil. Add the onions and fry until they start to soften, then gradually add the stock and keep reducing it down before adding more. Keep doing this until the onions become really caramelized, then with the very last bit of stock add the balsamic vinegar and cook until it has evaporated.

2. Reserve a couple of tablespoons of the fried onions and put the rest into a food processor with the chickpeas, the garlic, cumin, lemon juice and tahini, and pulse, adding a little of the chickpea liquid at a time until smooth. Taste and season with a pinch of salt.

3. Put the hummus into a bowl. Smooth over the top with a spatula, making some ridges in the hummus, top with the reserved caramelized onions, and drizzle over the olive oil.

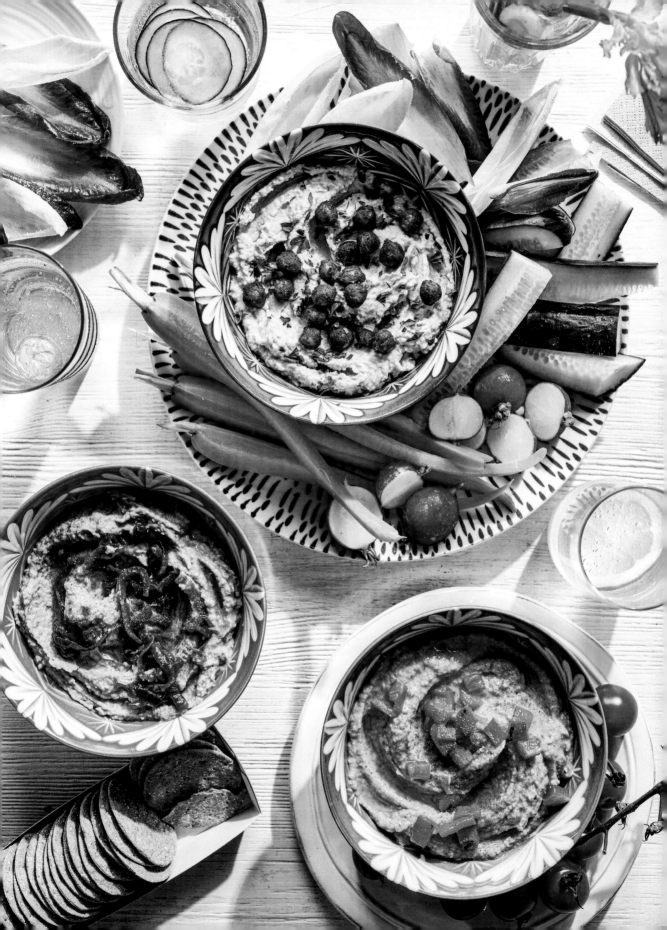

Roasted Red Pepper Hummus

KCALS: **92**

FAT: **3.6g**

SAT FAT: **0.5g**

CARBS: **8.7g**

SUGARS: **2.5g**

FIBRE: **4.0g**

PROTEIN: **4.2g**

SALT: **0.17g**

SERVES 6

2 red peppers
olive oil spray
1 x 400g (14oz) tin of
   chickpeas, drained,
   liquid reserved
2 garlic cloves, peeled
1 tablespoon tahini
½ teaspoon ground cumin
½ teaspoon paprika
   (plus an additional pinch)
juice of ½ a lemon
pinch of sea salt
1 teaspoon extra virgin
   olive oil
finely chopped fresh parsley

1. Preheat the oven to 220°C/200°C fan/425°F/gas 7.

2. Slice the peppers in half and remove all the pith and seeds. Place them on a baking tray, spray with olive oil, and roast for 30 minutes, until softened.

3. Remove from the oven, cover and let cool, then remove the skin from the peppers. Reserve half of one of the roasted red peppers and cut into small dice.

4. Put the rest of the peppers into a food processor. Add the chickpeas, the garlic, tahini, cumin, paprika and lemon juice, and pulse, adding some of the chickpea liquid until it has a smooth consistency. Taste and season with a pinch of sea salt.

5. Put the hummus into a bowl. Smooth over the top with a spatula, making some ridges in the hummus, and top with the diced reserved roasted red pepper, and an additional pinch of paprika. Drizzle over a teaspoon of olive oil and sprinkle with finely chopped parsley.

Cauliflower Rice 3 Ways

Cauliflower is probably one of my favourite vegetables. It makes a great low-carb dish and can be mashed and used as a substitute for mashed potatoes, or grated and used as rice. My favourite way to make basic cauliflower rice is by roasting it in the oven – roasting adds so much more flavour, and it's less messy when you grate it directly on to the tray you are baking it on. Here are three of my favourite versions of cauliflower rice. Try them as a side to one of the many delicious recipes in this book.

Special Fried Cauliflower Rice

SERVES 4

1 head of cauliflower
salt and freshly ground
    black pepper
olive oil spray
2 large eggs
1 onion, finely diced
1 carrot, finely diced
2 garlic cloves, crushed
120g (4oz) frozen peas
2 tablespoons soy sauce
1 teaspoon sesame oil
2 spring onions (scallions),
    chopped

Optional:
If not vegetarian, add some cubed ham, cooked chicken or cooked prawns (shrimp) at step 9 for some additional protein.

Gluten-free:
Use gluten-free soy sauce.

Freezing:
These cauliflower dishes are all good for freezing in handy portion-sized servings – to reheat, defrost in the fridge then warm through in the microwave or in a pan over a medium heat.

1. Preheat the oven to 180°C/160°C fan/350°F/gas 4. Line a large baking tray with parchment paper.

2. Coarsely grate the cauliflower directly on to the tray (or pulse it in a food processor if you prefer). Spread it out in an even layer on the tray and season with salt and freshly ground black pepper.

3. Spray over the top with olive oil and bake for about 30 minutes, until lightly charred on the edges. Remove from the oven and set aside.

4. Place a large frying pan over a medium–high heat and spray with olive oil.

5. Beat the eggs in a bowl and add to the pan, breaking them up with a wooden spoon as they start to cook. Remove from the pan and set aside.

6. Spray the pan with a little more olive oil.

7. Add the onion and carrot and fry until really softened, adding a pinch of salt.

8. Add the garlic and peas and fry for a further couple of minutes.

9. Add the cooked cauliflower rice, soy sauce and egg and mix to combine.

10. Stir in the sesame oil and spring onions, then season with salt and freshly ground black pepper.

11. Serve and enjoy!

161 Calories

KCALS: **161**

FAT: **5.2g**

SAT FAT: **1.1g**

CARBS: **15.4g**

SUGARS: **10.6g**

FIBRE: **6.0g**

PROTEIN: **10.1g**

SALT: **1.20g**

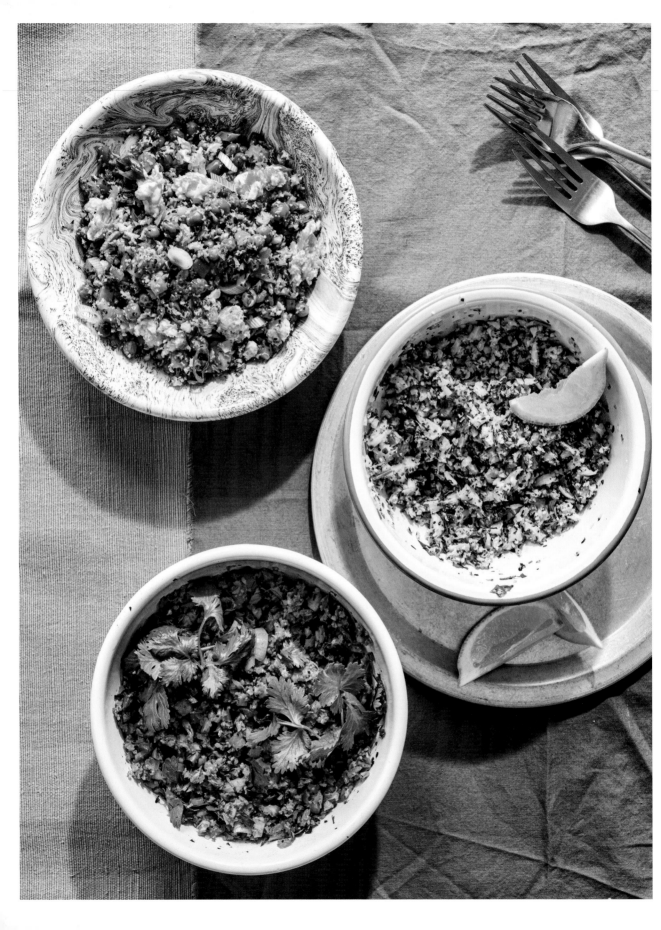

Garlic and Herb Cauliflower Rice   ❄

57 Calories

SERVES 4

1 head of cauliflower
3 garlic cloves, crushed
½ teaspoon fine salt
1 teaspoon dried basil
1 teaspoon dried oregano
½ teaspoon dried thyme
olive oil spray
1 tablespoon finely chopped
  fresh parsley
a little lemon juice

1. Preheat the oven to 180°C/160°C fan/350°F/gas 4. Line a large baking tray with parchment paper.

2. Coarsely grate the cauliflower directly on to the tray (or pulse it in a food processor if you prefer).

3. Add the garlic, salt, basil, oregano and thyme, and spread the cauliflower out in an even layer on the baking tray.

4. Spray the top with olive oil and bake for about 30 minutes, until lightly charred on the edges.

5. Remove from the oven, sprinkle with the chopped parsley, add a little squeeze of lemon juice, then toss it all on the tray.

KCALS: **57**

FAT: **0.9g**

SAT FAT: **0.2g**

CARBS: **6.9g**

SUGARS: **4.2g**

FIBRE: **3.0g**

PROTEIN: **4.0g**

SALT: **0.64g**

Spanish-style Cauliflower Rice   ❄

73 Calories

SERVES 4

1 head of cauliflower
salt and freshly ground
  black pepper
olive oil spray
1 small onion, finely diced
2 garlic cloves, crushed
2 tablespoons tomato purée
  (paste)
½ teaspoon dried oregano
1 teaspoon paprika
½ teaspoon ground cumin
pinch of red chilli flakes
120ml (4fl oz) chicken
  or vegetable stock
chopped fresh coriander
  (cilantro), or parsley if you
  don't like coriander

Vegetarian:
Use vegetable stock.

1. Preheat the oven to 180°C/160°C fan/350°F/gas 4. Line a large baking tray with parchment paper.

2. Coarsely grate the cauliflower directly on to the tray (or pulse it in a food processor if you prefer).

3. Season with salt and freshly ground black pepper and spread out in an even layer on the tray.

4. Spray the top with olive oil and bake for about 30 minutes, until lightly charred on the edges.

5. Place a large frying pan over a medium–high heat and spray with olive oil.

6. Add the onion and garlic and fry until softened.

7. Add the tomato purée, oregano and spices and gradually add the stock, reducing it down with each addition until you have a fragrant paste.

8. Add the cooked cauliflower rice and coriander, and toss until all combined.

9. Taste and season with salt and freshly ground black pepper.

10. Serve and enjoy!

KCALS: **73**

FAT: **1.3g**

SAT FAT: **0.2g**

CARBS: **8.9g**

SUGARS: **6.2g**

FIBRE: **3.9g**

PROTEIN: **4.5g**

SALT: **0.11g**

288
Calories

V

GF

KCALS
288

FAT
17.2g

SAT FAT
10.1g

CARBS
16.2g

SUGARS
9.4g

FIBRE
3.4g

PROTEIN
15.4g

SALT
0.88g

Cauliflower Cheese

SERVES 4

1 head of cauliflower,
    broken into florets
approx. 1.4l (2½ pints)
    vegetable or chicken stock
salt and freshly ground
    black pepper
3 spring onions (scallions),
    chopped (green part)
1 tablespoon butter
1 garlic clove, crushed
480ml (17fl oz) semi-
    skimmed milk
1½ tablespoons cornflour
    (cornstarch)
120g (4oz) strong mature
    Cheddar, grated
15g (½oz) golden
    breadcrumbs
    (optional)

Optional:
If not vegetarian, scatter
over some chopped cooked
bacon just before serving.

Gluten-free:
Use gluten-free breadcrumbs
if using.

Vegetarian:
Use vegetable stock.

Cauliflower cheese is one of those classic side dishes that is loved by many, and this lightened-up version doesn't disappoint. It still has all the cheesy goodness you expect, and can be used as a base recipe to build from. It's even more irresistible with some golden cooked bacon sprinkled on top, or some additional vegetables like sautéed leeks or broccoli.

1. Preheat the oven to 200°C/180°C fan/400°F/gas 6.

2. Put the cauliflower into a deep saucepan or frying pan and just cover with stock. Bring to the boil, then reduce the heat and simmer until tender (about 4–5 minutes). Drain the cauliflower and transfer to an ovenproof dish, season with salt and freshly ground black pepper and scatter over the spring onions.

3. Melt the butter in a small saucepan, then add the garlic and fry for 30 seconds, just to infuse the flavour.

4. Mix the milk with the cornflour and pour into the pan. Heat gently until it thickens (about 8 minutes), then add half the cheese and stir until melted.

5. Pour over the cauliflower, top with the remaining cheese, and sprinkle over the breadcrumbs if using.

6. Bake for 25 minutes, until golden.

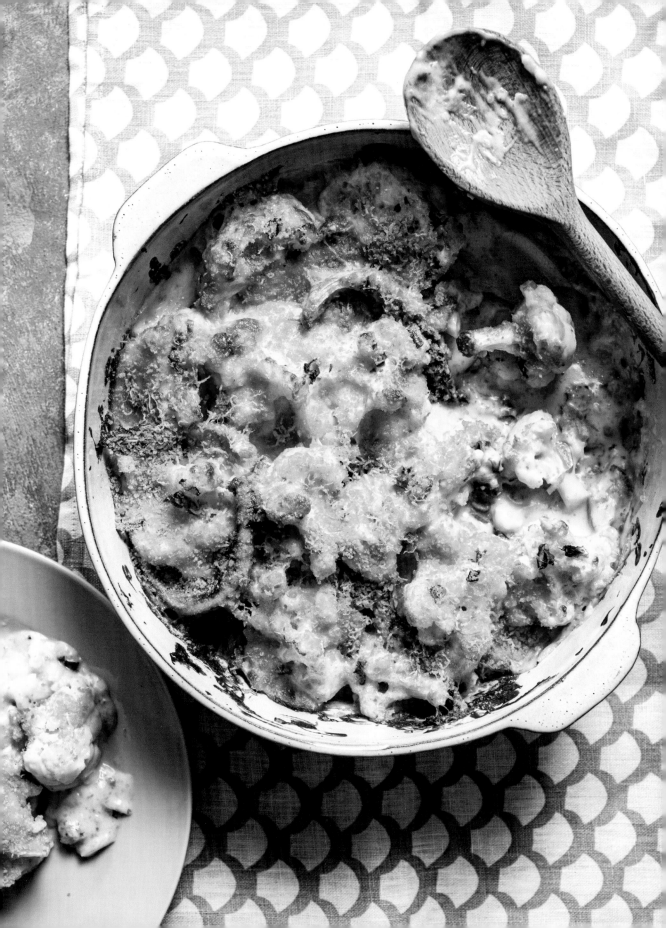

Potato Latkes

V

GF

DF

❄

KCALS
78

FAT
1.0g

SAT FAT
0.4g

CARBS
14.2g

SUGARS
1.1g

FIBRE
1.3g

PROTEIN
2.2g

SALT
0.20g

MAKES 15
(NUTRITIONAL ANALYSIS IS PER 3 LATKES)

800g (1lb 12oz) potatoes (use a floury variety)
1 onion (or spring onion/scallion)
½ teaspoon salt
½ teaspoon paprika
pinch of freshly ground black pepper
4 tablespoons cornflour (cornstarch)
2 large eggs
cooking oil spray (I use coconut or avocado)

Freezing:
To reheat after freezing, simply defrost in the fridge, then warm through in a frying pan over a medium heat.

Potato latkes traditionally combine grated potatoes, onion, matzo meal and seasonings, shallow-fried in oil to make them super golden and crispy. Typically they are served with apple sauce and soured cream (an amazing combination), but they are also nice paired with a variety of sides, or as a base for various toppings. I oven-bake my version to make them slightly healthier, and my family loves them with poached eggs.

1. Preheat the oven to 230°C/210°C fan/450°F/gas 8.

2. Peel and grate the potatoes, then squeeze out the excess liquid and blot with paper towels (this is important). Put the grated potatoes into a bowl.

3. Halve the onion and slice really thinly. Add this to the grated potato.

4. Add the salt, paprika and freshly ground black pepper and toss to coat.

5. Add the cornflour and eggs, and mix until all combined.

6. Line a large baking tray (you may need two if you don't have one big enough) with parchment paper and spray the paper with cooking oil.

7. Using an egg ring (or you can just roughly do it by hand), form 15 potato cakes. Flatten them down as well as you can on the tray (but don't place them too close together).

8. Spray the top with oil and bake in the oven for 40–45 minutes, carefully flipping them over halfway through the cooking time.

9. Serve with eggs or your favourite sides or toppings.

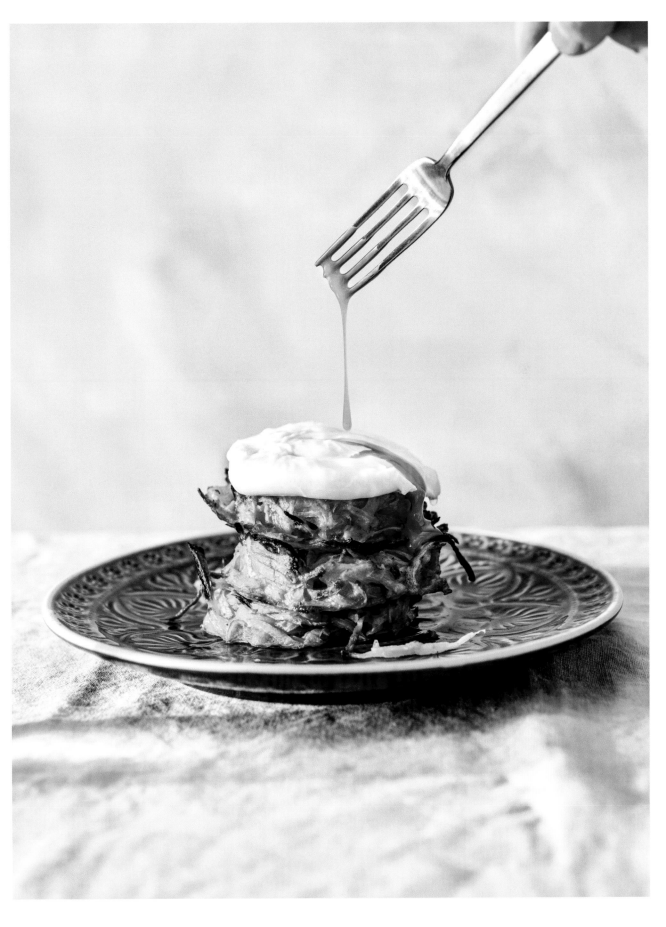

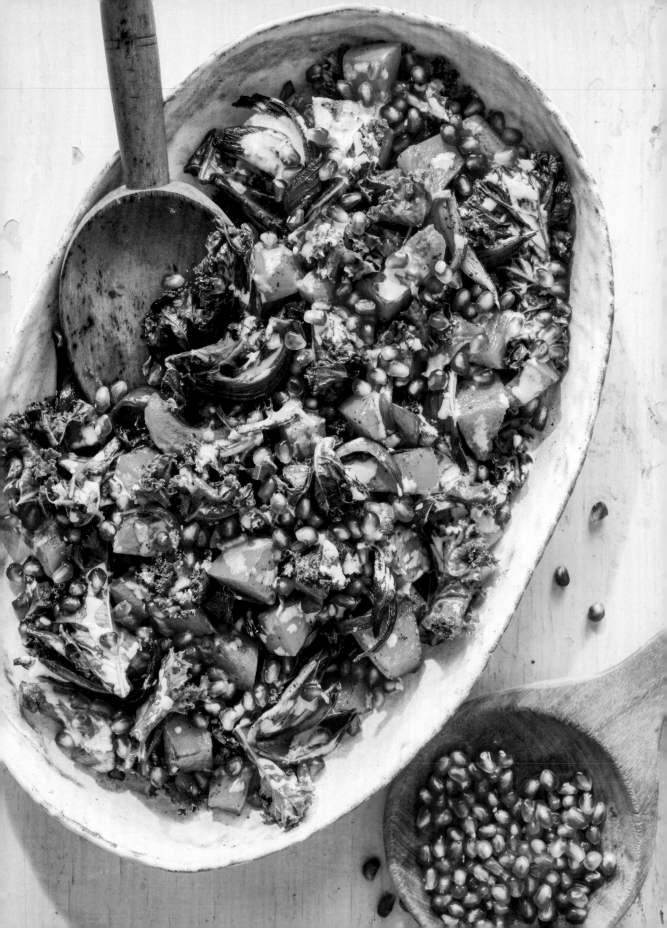

Sumac-roasted Butternut Squash with Tahini Dressing

SERVES 4

olive oil spray
700g (1lb 9oz) butternut
   squash, peeled and cubed
1 red onion, diced
1 teaspoon salt
2 teaspoons sumac
1 teaspoon paprika
1 garlic clove, crushed
4 big handfuls of kale,
   stalks removed, chopped
salt and freshly ground
   black pepper
1 pomegranate

For the tahini dressing:
1 tablespoon tahini
1 garlic clove, crushed
juice of ½ a lemon
pinch of salt
a little water if needed,
   to loosen dressing

Optional:
If not dairy-free, try this with
some crumbled feta over
the top. I also occasionally
like to add some tinned
chickpeas (for extra protein),
which I sauté in olive oil spray
with a good pinch of paprika,
garlic and salt.

This recipe combines two of my favourite vegetables, butternut squash and kale. The squash is roasted with the delicious flavours of sumac and paprika, and the kale is lightly sautéed with garlic. It's all finished off with fresh pomegranate seeds, which add a sweet crunch, with a light tahini dressing for additional flavour.

1. Preheat the oven to 200°C/180°C fan/400°F/gas 6. Line a baking tray with parchment paper and spray the paper with olive oil.

2. Put the dressing ingredients into a bowl and whisk until combined.

3. Put the butternut squash, onion and seasonings on the lined tray and toss to coat. Then spread them out in a thin, even layer on the tray, making sure they're not crammed too close together.

4. Spray the top with olive oil and bake for 35–40 minutes, until light golden and softened.

5. Place a frying pan over a medium–high heat and spray with olive oil. Add the garlic to the pan and cook for 30 seconds, just to infuse the flavour, then add the kale with a good pinch of salt and some freshly ground black pepper and cook until it slightly wilts down (be careful not to let it burn). Transfer to a large plate.

6. Top with the roasted squash, scatter over the pomegranate seeds and drizzle with the tahini dressing. Enjoy!

KCALS
177

FAT
4.5g

SAT FAT
0.5g

CARBS
24.7g

SUGARS
17.6g

FIBRE
8.6g

PROTEIN
5.1g

SALT
1.33g

Jalapeño Poppers

KCALS
137

FAT
5.6g

SAT FAT
3.2g

CARBS
9.7g

SUGARS
4.9g

FIBRE
1.5g

PROTEIN
11.3g

SALT
0.74g

SERVES 3

6 large jalapeños (if your
   jalapeños are small,
   you may need about 9)
120g (4oz) low-fat
   cream cheese
80g (3oz) fat-free
   Greek yoghurt
pinch of salt
½ teaspoon onion powder
½ teaspoon garlic powder
1 tablespoon chopped
   fresh chives
30g (1oz) Cheddar,
   finely grated
20g (¾oz) panko
   breadcrumbs
olive oil spray

Gluten-free:
Use gluten-free breadcrumbs
instead of panko.

Additions:
Add some diced cooked
bacon to your cream cheese/
yoghurt mix.

If there is one little side/appetizer I adore, it's jalapeño poppers. That taste of spicy cream cheese, deep-fried to perfection, is just heavenly, but as with anything deep-fried, the calories can be a little excessive. Instead, for my lighter take, I bake these in the oven with a cream cheese and Greek yoghurt filling, topped with golden panko breadcrumbs and Cheddar.

1. Preheat the oven to 200°C/180°C fan/400°F/gas 6. Line a baking tray with foil.

2. Cut the jalapeños in half and remove the seeds and white pith (be careful not to touch your eyes, or wear gloves).

3. In a bowl mix together the cream cheese and Greek yoghurt with the salt, the onion powder, garlic powder and chives.

4. Spoon the mixture into the jalapeños and place them on the lined baking tray.

5. Put the Cheddar and panko into a bowl, and crumble up with your hands so you have small crumbs of cheese and breadcrumbs.

6. Sprinkle the crumbs on top of the cream cheese and spray with olive oil.

7. Bake in the oven for about 25–30 minutes, until golden on top.

8. Allow to slightly cool before eating!

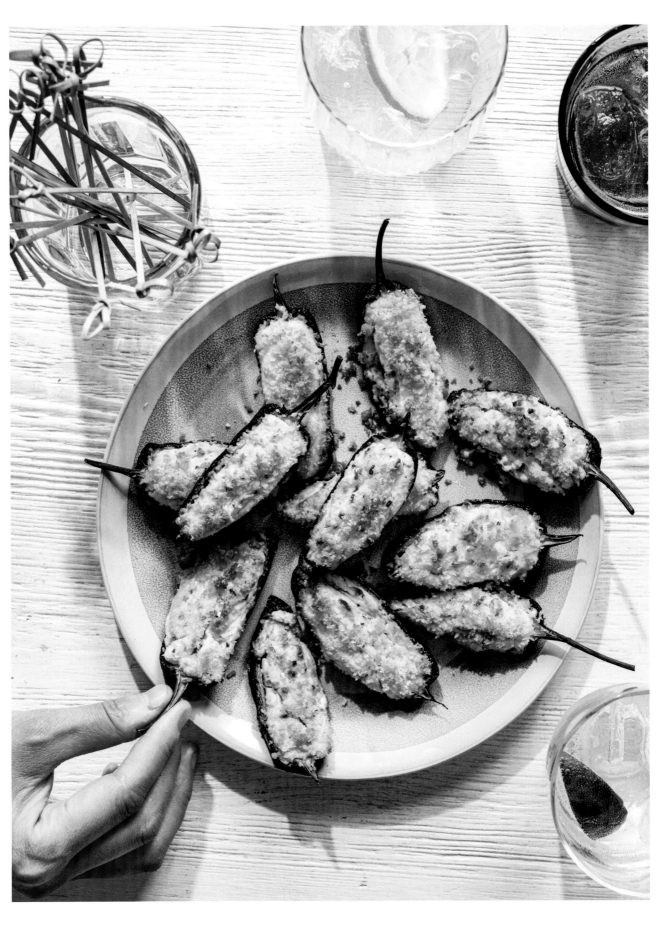

165
Calories

V

GF

KCALS
165

FAT
8.2g

SAT FAT
4.6g

CARBS
6.4g

SUGARS
4.1g

FIBRE
5.1g

PROTEIN
14.0g

SALT
0.55g

Smashed Cheddar Broccoli with Ranch Dip

SERVES 4

600g (1lb 5oz) broccoli
   florets
olive oil spray
1 teaspoon smoked paprika
½ teaspoon garlic powder
pinch of salt and freshly
   ground black pepper
80g (3oz) Cheddar, grated

For the ranch dip:
120g (4oz) fat-free
   Greek yoghurt
1 tablespoon milk
½ tablespoon lemon juice
1 teaspoon maple syrup
   (optional)
½ teaspoon garlic powder
½ teaspoon onion powder
½ teaspoon dried parsley
½ teaspoon dried dill
pinch of salt and freshly
   ground black pepper

Tip:
The ranch dip is perfect
as a dressing for salad
or as a dip for chicken,
veggies and more.

Do you struggle to get a decent amount of veggies into your meals? Then this is just the recipe for you. Even my kids will devour these cheesy Cheddar-smashed morsels of roasted broccoli, with the healthy Greek yoghurt ranch dip on the side. You can also enjoy the dip as a dressing to drizzle over salads.

1. Preheat the oven to 220°C/200°C fan/425°F/gas 7. Line a baking tray with parchment paper.

2. Bring a large saucepan of water to the boil. Drop in the broccoli just for 1 minute, until it turns bright green, then remove and transfer to the lined baking tray.

3. Spray with olive oil, add the paprika, garlic powder and a pinch of salt and freshly ground black pepper, and toss to coat.

4. Spread out on the baking tray, spray the top with a little more olive oil, and roast for 15 minutes.

5. Remove the tray from the oven and squish the broccoli down slightly with a fork, then sprinkle the grated Cheddar on top of each smashed floret.

6. Place back in the oven and bake for 15 minutes, until the cheese is melted and golden.

7. Mix all the ingredients for the ranch dip together in a bowl, and serve with the broccoli.

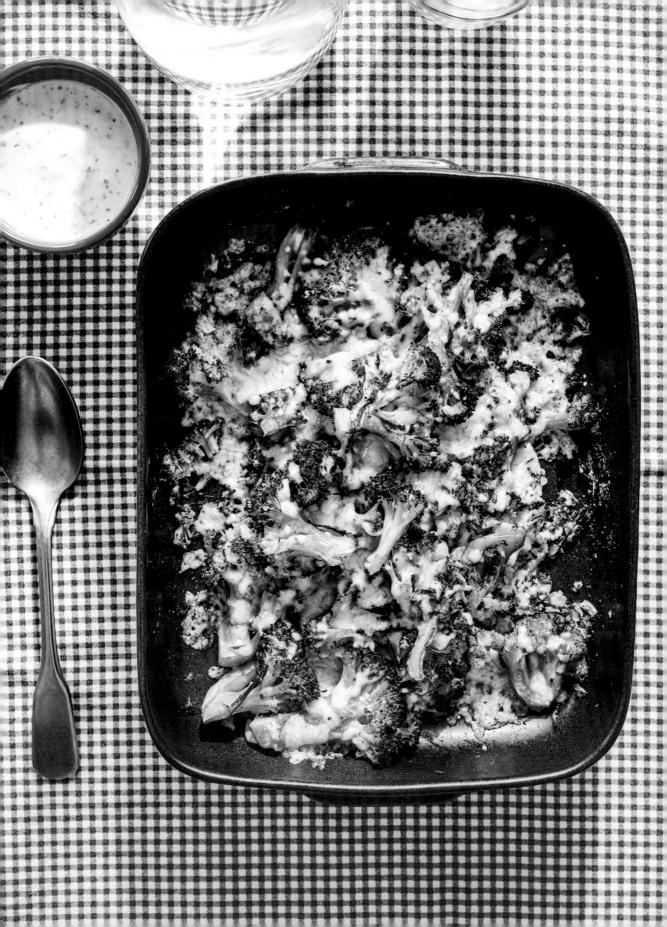

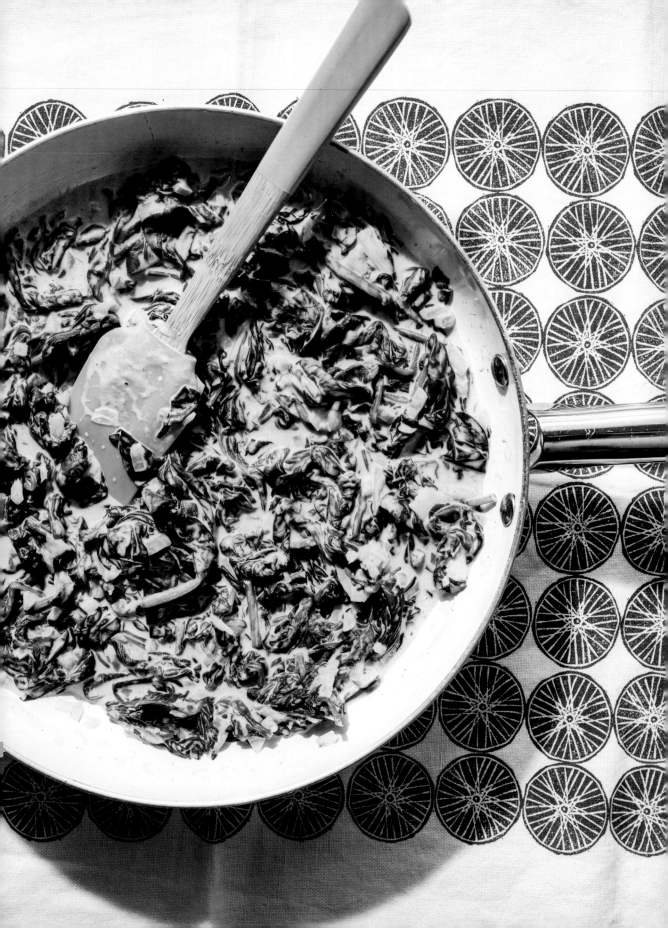

Creamed Spinach

SERVES 4

olive oil spray
455g (1lb) spinach
1 small onion, finely chopped
2 garlic cloves, crushed
300ml (10fl oz) vegetable
   or chicken stock
pinch of cayenne pepper
pinch of paprika
100g (3½oz) light
   cream cheese
30g (1½oz) Parmesan
   or vegetarian Italian-style
   hard cheese, grated
salt and freshly ground
   black pepper

Vegetarian:
Use vegetable stock
and vegetarian Italian-style
hard cheese.

Serving suggestions:
Great served with chicken,
fish or steak.

This addictive recipe is the ultimate vegetable side dish to accompany a variety of main meals. Sautéed fresh spinach in a lighter creamy sauce – simple to make and ready in minutes.

1. Spray a frying pan placed over a medium–high heat with some olive oil.

2. Add the spinach (in 2 batches) and cook until wilted down. Transfer to a plate.

3. Spray the pan with a little more olive oil, then add the onion and garlic and fry until lightly golden. Take about a third of the stock and keep adding a little at a time to the pan, reducing it down as you do, until the stock is gone and the onion and garlic have really softened.

4. Add a pinch of cayenne and paprika.

5. Add the remaining stock and the cream cheese and stir until the cheese has all melted. Add the Parmesan and stir until the sauce has slightly thickened.

6. Return the spinach to the pan and stir until it is all creamy. Taste and season with salt and freshly ground black pepper.

7. Enjoy!

KCALS
100

FAT
4.5g

SAT FAT
2.2g

CARBS
3.2g

SUGARS
2.3g

FIBRE
1.8g

PROTEIN
10.6g

SALT
0.80g

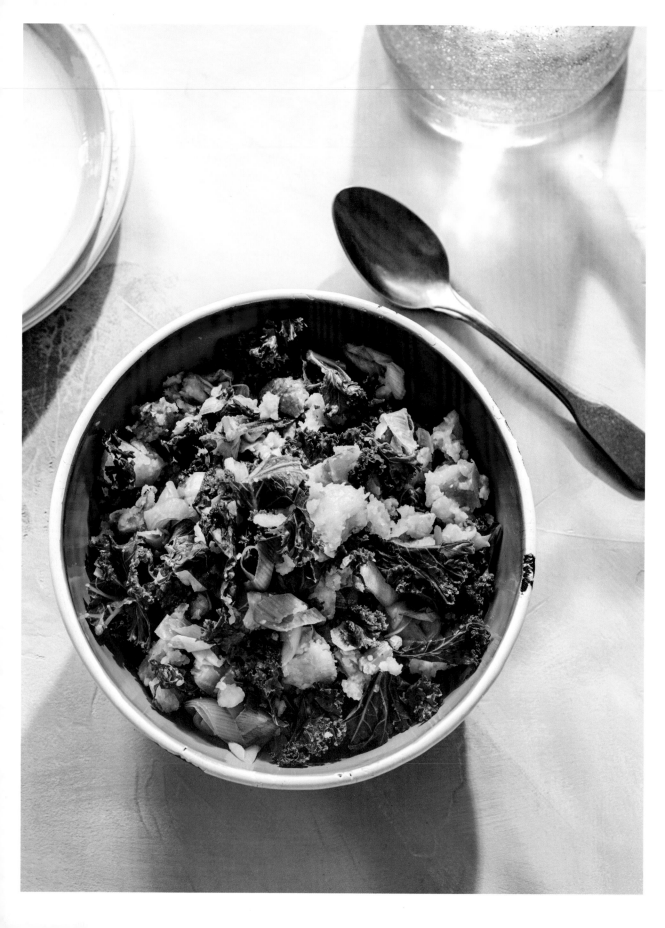

Rustic Kale and Leek Potato Mash

SERVES 4

olive oil spray
3 garlic cloves, crushed
1 leek, trimmed, sliced and
    washed
200g (7oz) kale, stalks
    removed, roughly chopped
480ml (17fl oz) vegetable or
    chicken stock
500g (1lb 2oz) baby potatoes
    in skins (waxy variety),
    halved
salt and freshly ground
    black pepper

Vegetarian:
Use vegetable stock.

Optional:
Serve with a knob of butter
on top.

Freezing:
To reheat after freezing,
simply defrost in the fridge,
then warm through in the
microwave or in a non-stick
frying pan over a medium
heat.

If you love colcannon, you will love my twist on this classic side dish, made with baby potatoes roughly mashed in their skins, with sautéed leeks, garlic and kale.

1. Place a frying pan over a medium–high heat and spray with olive oil.

2. Add the garlic and fry for a minute to soften and infuse (be careful not to let it burn).

3. Add the leek and kale and a quarter of the stock and cook until the stock has evaporated and the kale and leek are softened. Remove from the pan and set aside.

4. Put the halved potatoes flesh side down into the same pan, add the rest of the stock, bring to the boil, then cover and reduce the heat to medium. Simmer for 15 minutes until the potatoes are tender, then remove the lid and turn the heat back up.

5. Spray the potatoes with olive oil and add a little pinch of salt and freshly ground black pepper, then start to roughly mash them in the pan while the remaining stock evaporates.

6. Return the kale and leek to the pan and mix until all combined, and serve.

KCALS
143

FAT
1.6g

SAT FAT
0.2g

CARBS
23.9g

SUGARS
3.4g

FIBRE
6.0g

PROTEIN
5.1g

SALT
0.36g

Indian Roasted Cauliflower Pilau Rice

KCALS
244

FAT
5.8g

SAT FAT
1.1g

CARBS
36.7g

SUGARS
6.4g

FIBRE
3.4g

PROTEIN
9.5g

SALT
0.48g

SERVES 6

For the cauliflower:
1 head of cauliflower,
    sliced into 1cm (½ inch)
    steaks, then broken into
    smaller pieces
cooking oil spray
1 teaspoon ground cumin
1 teaspoon turmeric
salt and freshly ground
    black pepper

For the rice:
30 raw cashews
salt
1 small onion, quartered
    and thinly sliced
1 teaspoon cumin seeds
2 garlic cloves, crushed
1 teaspoon grated fresh
    ginger
½ teaspoon turmeric
200g (7oz) basmati rice,
    rinsed
1 green chilli, sliced in half
20g (¾oz) sultanas
4 cardamom pods
4 cloves
450ml (16fl oz) chicken stock
chopped fresh coriander
    (cilantro)

**The ideal side to an Indian-style main, this pilau rice is
beautifully flavoured with Indian spices and is combined
with roasted spiced cauliflower.**

1. Preheat the oven to 200°C/180°C fan/400°F/gas 6.

2. Place the cauliflower on a baking tray lined with parchment
paper, spray with cooking oil, sprinkle with the cumin, turmeric
and a pinch of salt and freshly ground black pepper, then carefully
toss on the tray to coat.

3. Bake until golden and slightly charred – about 20 minutes.

4. While the cauliflower is roasting, spray a frying pan with cooking
oil, add the cashews and a pinch of salt, and toast in the pan for
about 3 minutes, stirring often, until golden. Remove from the pan
and set aside.

5. Spray the frying pan again, add the onion and fry until golden/
translucent, add the cumin seeds and fry for a further minute,
then add the garlic, ginger and turmeric and mix to coat, adding
a little water to prevent burning.

6. Add the rice and stir in the pan until it is mixed with the onion
and turns a golden yellow colour, then add the green chilli, sultanas,
cardamom pods, cloves and stock. Bring to the boil, then reduce the
heat, cover the pan and simmer until the stock is just about absorbed.
Turn off the heat, but leave lidded for 12 minutes (don't touch).

7. After 12 minutes, remove the lid and fluff up the rice. Transfer it
to a large plate, toss with the roasted cauliflower, and sprinkle with
the toasted cashews and some fresh coriander.

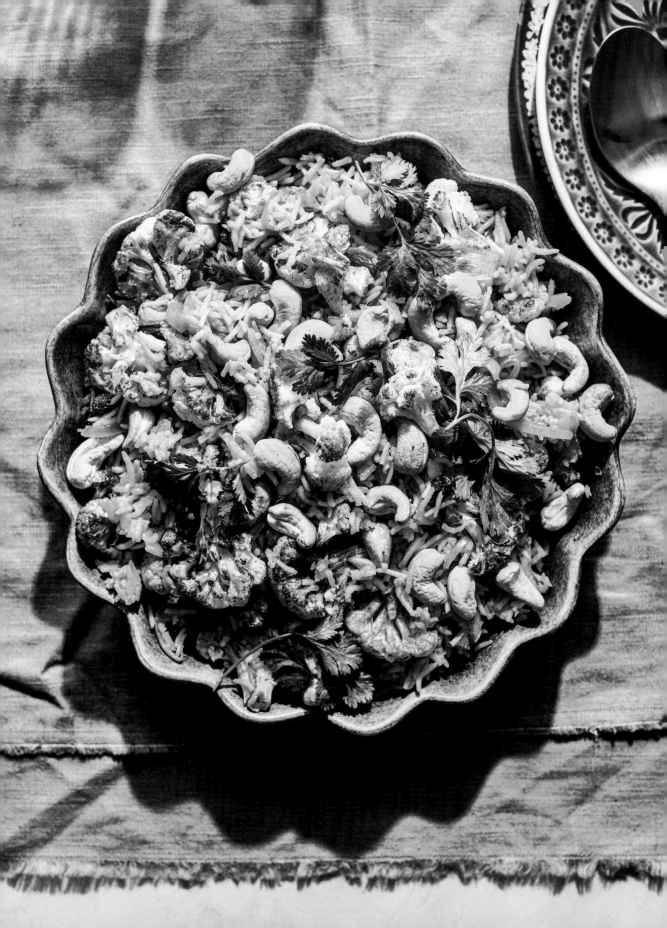

Desserts

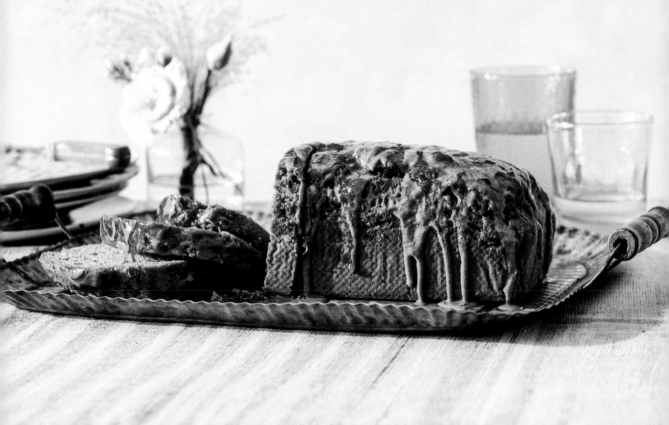

Coconut and Lemon
Muffins

Raspberry,
Pear and White
Chocolate Pies

Chocolate Cake

Strawberry Jelly
Chocolate Ice Lollies

Apple Berry Cream
Cheese Filo Tart

Hot Banana
Pudding Custard
with Cookie Crumb

Peanut Butter
Jelly Banana Bread

No-bake Strawberry
Cheesecakes

Chocolate Orange
Rice Pudding

Oaty Apple
Crumble

Cinnamon Sugar
Pecan-baked
Bananas with
Greek Yoghurt

148
Calories

Coconut and Lemon Muffins

KCALS
148

FAT
5.3g

SAT FAT
3.5g

CARBS
18.7g

SUGARS
9.7g

FIBRE
1.8g

PROTEIN
4.8g

SALT
0.42g

MAKES 10 MUFFINS

100g (3½oz) plain
   (all-purpose) flour
30g (1oz) coconut flour
1 teaspoon baking powder
½ teaspoon bicarbonate
   of soda (baking soda)
pinch of salt
180g (6oz) cottage cheese
2 large eggs
1 teaspoon coconut extract
1 teaspoon lemon extract
a little lemon zest
4 tablespoons maple syrup
2 tablespoons coconut oil,
   melted
4 tablespoons granulated
   sweetener
cooking oil spray

For the glaze:
a little fresh lemon juice
40g (1½oz) icing sugar
   (confectioners' sugar)
5g (⅛oz) unsweetened
   shredded coconut

Freezing:
Freeze after step 7, once cool.
To eat, defrost the muffins
at room temperature, then
make the icing and drizzle
over the top before serving.

Two of my favourite flavours for cake combined together in these yummy coconut and lemon muffins, finished off with a light lemon glaze and a scattering of shredded coconut.

1. Preheat the oven to 180°C/160°C fan/350°F/gas 4.

2. Combine the flours, baking powder, bicarbonate of soda and salt in a bowl.

3. Put the cottage cheese and eggs into a blender and blend until smooth.

4. Transfer to a bowl and mix in the coconut extract, lemon extract, lemon zest, maple syrup, melted coconut oil and granulated sweetener.

5. Add this to the flour mixture and combine.

6. Spoon into 10 parchment muffin cases lightly misted with cooking oil spray.

7. Bake in the oven for 30 minutes (a skewer inserted into the centre should come out clean).

8. Allow to cool, then add lemon juice a little at a time to the icing sugar until glaze-like and drizzle over the top of the muffins. Finish with the shredded coconut, then serve with a cuppa.

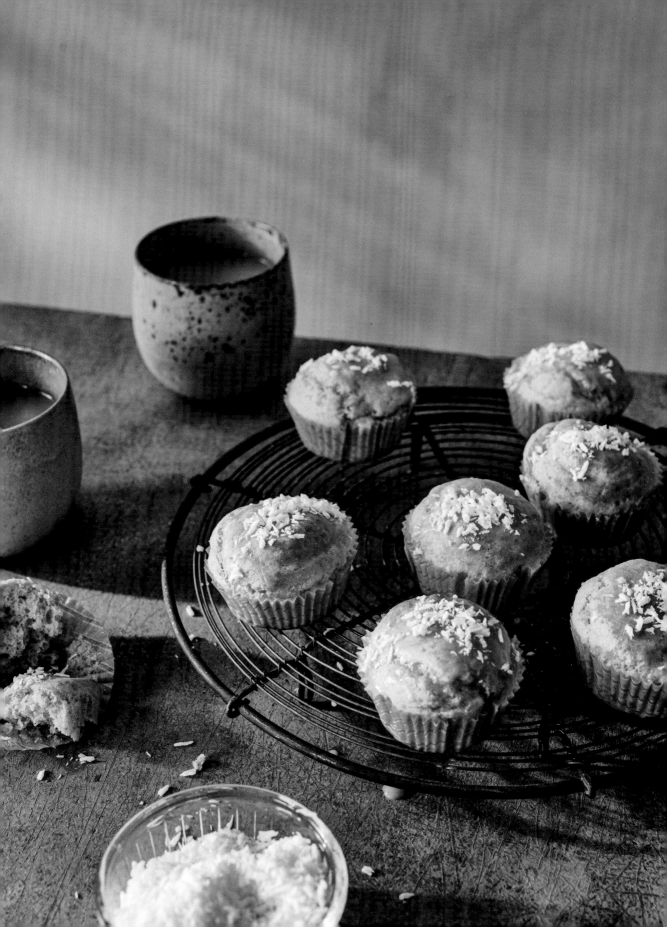

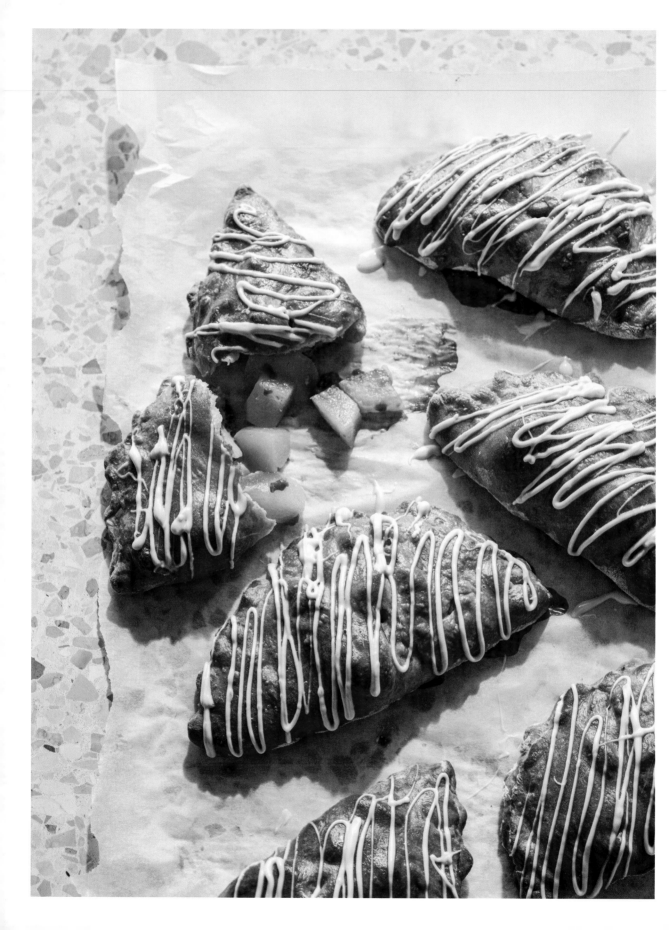

Raspberry, Pear and White Chocolate Pies

MAKES 6 PIES

120g (4oz) plain
  (all-purpose) flour
1½ teaspoons baking powder
1 tablespoon granulated
  sweetener
140g (5oz) fat-free
  Greek yoghurt
1 egg
coconut oil spray

For the filling:
1 pear (approx. 140g/5oz)
30g (1oz) raspberries
1 tablespoon white
  chocolate chips

Variation:
Try different fruit fillings,
and if you don't like white
chocolate you can also
use milk or dark chocolate
for these.

These pies are such a satisfying swet treat, and use a healthy Greek yoghurt dough instead of high-calorie pastry. Whenever I make a batch of these, they are gone in seconds.

1. Preheat the oven to 200°C/180°C fan/400°F/gas 6.

2. Set aside about ¾ tablespoon of the flour for dusting. Put the remaining flour into a bowl with the baking powder and sweetener and mix to combine.

3. Add the yoghurt, then use a wooden spoon or silicone spatula to bring the dough together. Once this starts to happen you can knead with your hands until the sides of the bowl are clear and you have one big dough ball.

4. Divide the dough into 6 equal-sized balls.

5. Beat the egg in a bowl.

6. Dust a surface with flour, add one ball of the dough, and lightly dust over the top with flour. Place a square of parchment paper on top of the dough ball and flatten down with a heavy saucepan, then roll flat (rotating and flipping the dough as you roll) until you have a circle about 14cm (5½ inches) across.

7. Peel and chop the pear and mix with the raspberries. Spoon one-sixth of the pear/raspberry mix on to one side of the circle, brush the edge of that side with egg wash, then fold over so you have a half-circle shape and seal all around the edges by crimping them together with a fork. Make a steam hole by piercing the top with a fork, then brush all over the top with egg wash. Repeat with the remaining balls of dough.

8. Spray the tops of the pies with the oil, then bake for 20 minutes, until golden.

9. Remove from the oven and allow to cool slightly.

10. Put the chocolate chips into a bowl and melt them in the microwave (about 30 seconds). Put the melted chocolate into a ziplock bag and push it all to one corner, then snip off the corner and pipe the chocolate across the top of the pies.

KCALS
129

FAT
2.1g

SAT FAT
0.9g

CARBS
209g

SUGARS
5.1g

FIBRE
1.6g

PROTEIN
5.9g

SALT
0.36g

163 Calories

Chocolate Cake

KCALS
163

FAT
5.2g

SAT FAT
3.4g

CARBS
24.2g

SUGARS
9.1g

FIBRE
1.6g

PROTEIN
3.6g

SALT
0.34g

MAKES 9 SQUARES

160g (5½oz) plain
  (all-purpose) flour
1 teaspoon baking powder
½ teaspoon bicarbonate
  of soda (baking soda)
pinch of salt
15g (½oz) cocoa powder
130g (4½oz) banana, mashed
4 tablespoons maple syrup
2 tablespoons coconut oil
  or butter (melted)
120ml (4fl oz) chocolate
  almond milk
1 large egg
1 teaspoon vanilla extract

For the chocolate milk drizzle:
60ml (2fl oz) chocolate
  almond milk
30g (1oz) milk or dark
  chocolate chips

Dairy-free:
Ensure you use dark rather
than milk chocolate.

Freezing:
To eat after freezing, simply
defrost in the fridge. You
could warm the cake through
in the microwave if you like.

If you can't get enough of chocolate, this delicious cake will satisfy all your cravings. The final chocolate milk drizzle keeps the cake lovely and moist. Good on its own with a cuppa, or served with some berries.

1. Combine the dry ingredients in a bowl.

2. Combine the wet ingredients in a second bowl.

3. Fold the wet ingredients into the dry ingredients.

4. Preheat the oven to 180°C/160°C fan/350°F/gas 4, and line a 20cm (8 inch) square cake tin with parchment paper.

5. Put the mixture into the lined tin.

6. Bake for 20–25 minutes, until a skewer inserted into the centre comes out clean.

7. Remove from the oven and poke holes all over the top of cake with a skewer.

8. To make the drizzle, put the chocolate almond milk into a small saucepan and bring to a slow bubble.

9. Remove from the heat and stir in the chocolate chips until melted.

10. Pour this all over the top of the cake.

11. Enjoy as is, or serve with some berries and light aerosol cream for a decadent dessert.

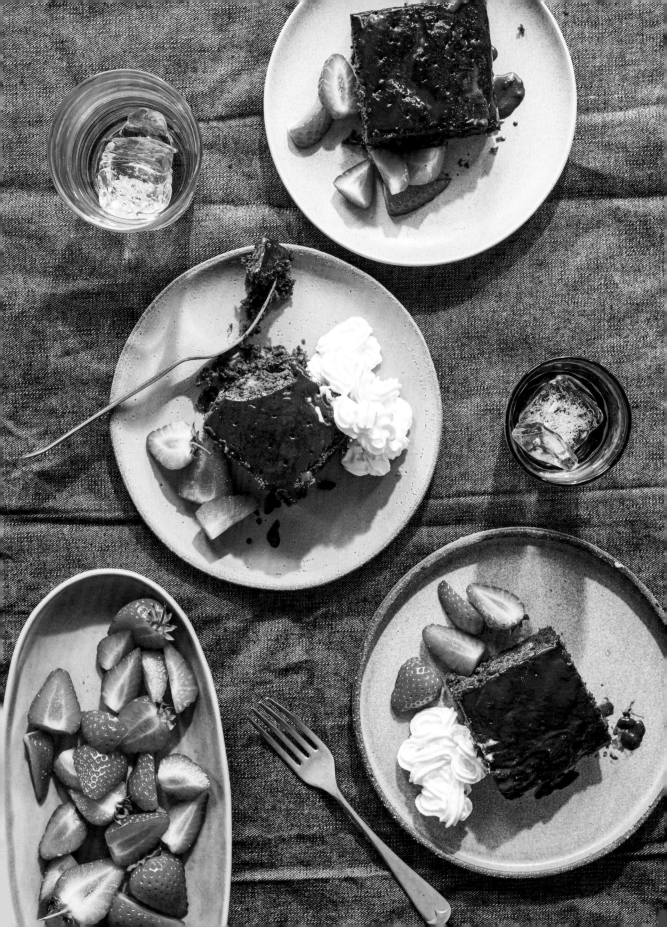

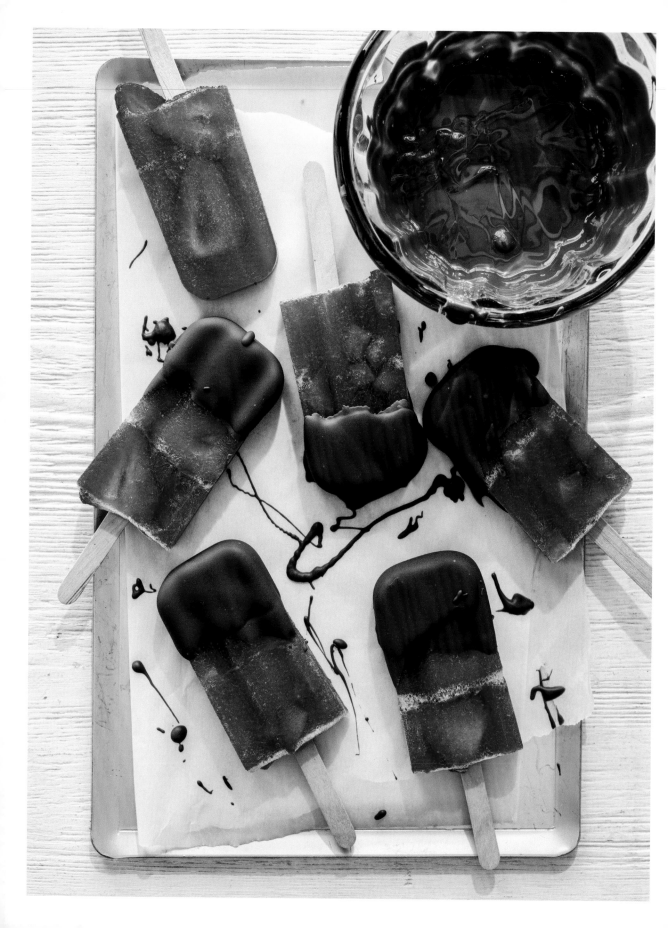

Strawberry Jelly Chocolate Ice Lollies

MAKES 6 ICE LOLLIES

1 carton of sugar-free
   strawberry jelly
240ml (9fl oz) hot water
240ml (9fl oz) apple juice
approx. 20 small
   strawberries, chopped
150g (5½oz) milk chocolate
1 teaspoon coconut oil

Swap:
Try different jelly flavours for
more variations on these.

These strawberry jelly chocolate ice lollies are the ultimate cooling summertime treat. They are super refreshing, and are super easy to make. They can also be varied in flavour by swapping the jelly for other flavours.

1. Dissolve the jelly in the hot water, then add the apple juice.

2. Pour into the ice lolly moulds (but only fill them two-thirds of the way up), then drop fresh strawberries into the moulds, pushing them down with the end of a spoon.

3. Place in the freezer until fully frozen.

4. Once frozen, remove the lollies from the moulds (you may need to run the moulds under water until easy to remove) and place on a baking tray lined with parchment paper. Pop them back into the freezer (they must be fully frozen before dipping, otherwise the chocolate won't stick).

5. Put the chocolate and coconut oil into a bowl and microwave at 20-second intervals until all melted.

6. One at a time, dip the ends of the lollies into the chocolate so that just a third of each lolly is dipped. Ensure you allow any excess to drip off. Then put back on the parchment paper and freeze until set. Once fully frozen, you can put them into individual bags or a tub.

7. You will have some melted chocolate left over (you need the extra otherwise it is not deep enough to dip). Store the leftover chocolate in a container – it makes a great chocolate magic dip for ice cream or lollies.

KCALS
177

FAT
9.0g

SAT FAT
5.2g

CARBS
19.8g

SUGARS
19.8g

FIBRE
2.1g

PROTEIN
13.2g

SALT
0.13g

Apple Berry Cream Cheese Filo Tart

(V)

SERVES 4

300g (10½oz) apples,
  peeled and sliced
5 tablespoons orange juice
1 tablespoon brown sugar
2 large eggs
cooking oil spray
4 sheets of filo pastry
120g (4oz) low-fat
  cream cheese
a little orange zest
2 tablespoons granulated
  sweetener
1 teaspoon vanilla extract
140g (5oz) frozen berries,
  defrosted
1 teaspoon icing sugar
  (confectioners' sugar),
  for dusting

Variations:
Try different fruit fillings
and if you don't like white
chocolate you can also
use milk or dark chocolate
for these.

KCALS	**272**
FAT	**5.6g**
SAT FAT	**1.7g**
CARBS	**41.8g**
SUGARS	**19.9g**
FIBRE	**3.7g**
PROTEIN	**11.2g**
SALT	**0.66g**

Made the delicious healthier chicken pot pie (page 98) or the garlic, mushroom, onion and jalapeño filo tart (page 184) and wondering what you can make with the leftover filo? This apple berry cream cheese filo tart is a must. Flaky golden filo pastry is topped with cream cheese and fruit. Yum!

1. Put the apples, 4 tablespoons of the orange juice and the brown sugar into a saucepan and cook until the apples are softened and all the liquid has been cooked off.

2. Beat one of the eggs in a bowl.

3. Line a 33 x 24cm (13 x 9½ inch) baking tray with parchment paper and spray the paper with cooking oil.

4. Lay the 4 sheets of filo on the baking tray, one on top of the other. Then roughly fold over the edges to make a large rectangular tart shape.

5. Spray the top with cooking oil and bake in the oven for about 6–8 minutes, just until lightly golden.

6. Remove from the oven and brush with the beaten egg.

7. In a bowl whisk the other egg with the cream cheese, the remaining tablespoon of orange juice, the orange zest, sweetener and vanilla.

8. Spread this mixture over the tart in an even layer.

9. Top with the apples and place back in the oven for 15–20 minutes. The tart should be lovely and golden and the cream cheese mixture set.

10. Allow to cool slightly. Then scatter over the slightly defrosted berries (make sure to not add too much of the juice).

11. Dust with the icing sugar, slice and serve.

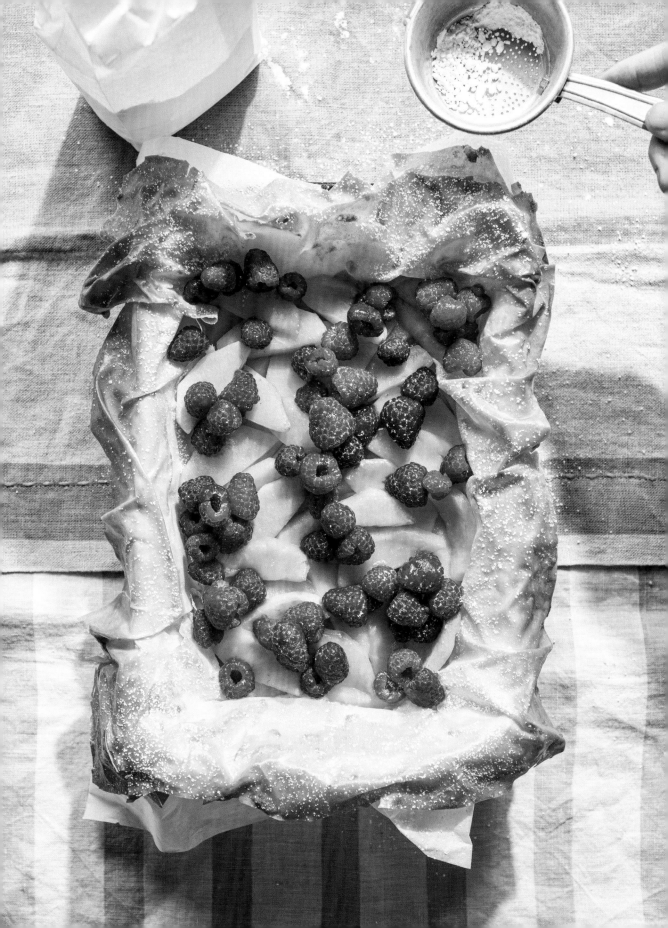

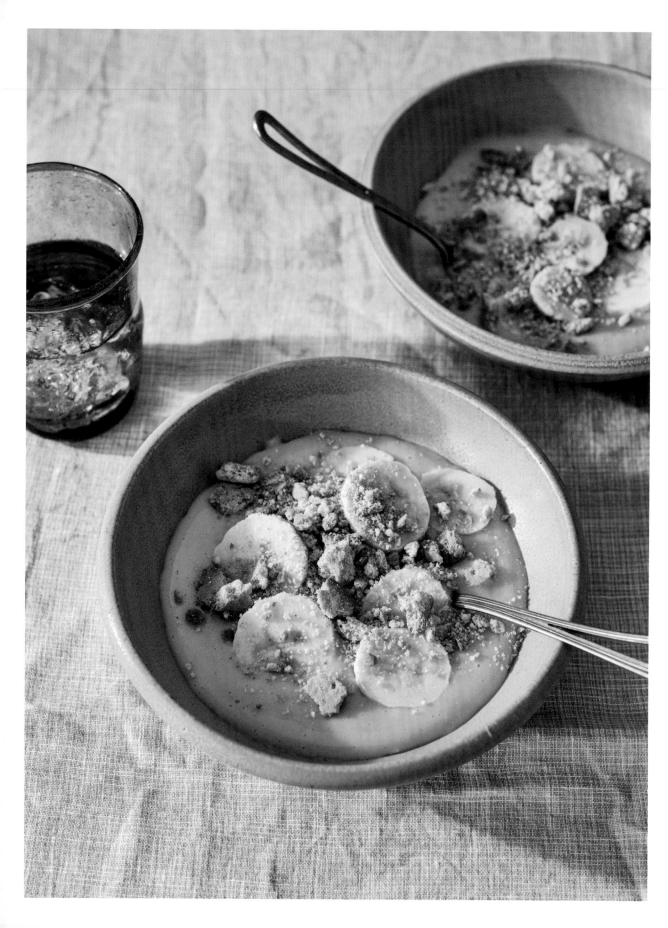

Hot Banana Pudding Custard with Cookie Crumb

SERVES 2

240ml (9fl oz) semi-skimmed milk

2 tablespoons maple syrup

1½ tablespoons cornflour (cornstarch)

1 teaspoon vanilla extract

1 egg yolk

1 large banana, sliced

2 reduced-fat digestives, crumbled (or other biscuit/cookie of your choice)

Gluten-free:
Use gluten-free cornflour and biscuits.

Anyone remember those hot puddings from the '80s (showing my age here) that you used to get in a sachet, with the cookie crunch to sprinkle on top, which came in lemon or banana flavours? For me they are vivid childhood dessert memories, along with gypsy tart, and even to this day I still get cravings... so guess what I did? Came up with my own version. These are a pure comfort treat in a bowl, and super easy to make.

1. Combine the milk, maple syrup, cornflour and vanilla in a bowl.

2. Transfer to a saucepan and gently heat, stirring until the mixture thickens.

3. Remove from the heat and quickly stir in the egg yolk.

4. Add half the sliced banana and stir to combine. Divide between two bowls, top with the rest of the banana, and sprinkle over the crumbled digestives.

5. Enjoy!

KCALS
286

FAT
6.8g

SAT FAT
2.7g

CARBS
47.3g

SUGARS
28.4g

FIBRE
1.3g

PROTEIN
7.1g

SALT
0.30g

Peanut Butter Jelly Banana Bread

V

DF

❄

KCALS
150

FAT
5.1g

SAT FAT
1.3g

CARBS
19.9g

SUGARS
4.1g

FIBRE
1.4g

PROTEIN
5.1g

SALT
0.42g

MAKES 10 SLICES

160g (6oz) plain flour
(all-purpose flour)
1 teaspoon baking powder
½ teaspoon bicarbonate
of soda (baking soda)
pinch of salt
180g (6oz) bananas
4 tablespoons natural
peanut butter
6 tablespoons granulated
brown sweetener
1 teaspoon vanilla extract
2 eggs

For the top:
1 tablespoon peanut butter
2 tablespoons reduced-sugar
strawberry jam
1 tablespoon water

Freezing:
To eat after freezing, simply
defrost in the fridge. You
could warm the bread
through in the microwave if
you like.

This is a recipe inspired by my children. I regularly make banana
bread with chocolate chips, which they love, so I asked them –
if I made a different kind of banana bread, which flavours would
be their favourite? Of course, with them both loving peanut
butter and jelly sandwiches, you can guess what they answered.
So here it is, and we have to thank them for it, as it's just the
best combo ever.

1. Preheat the oven to 180°C/160°C fan/350°F/gas 4.

2. Combine the flour, baking powder, bicarbonate of soda and salt
in a bowl.

3. In another bowl mash the bananas, then add the peanut butter,
sweetener, vanilla and eggs.

4. Fold the banana mixture into the flour mixture until combined.

5. Grease a loaf tin (I prefer to line it with parchment paper) and
spoon in the batter.

6. Bake in the oven for 40 minutes, until a skewer inserted into the
centre comes out clean.

7. Remove from the oven and leave to cool for about 15 minutes.

8. Microwave the peanut butter at 10-second intervals until runny,
then drizzle over the top of the loaf.

9. Microwave the jam at 10-second intervals with the water until
runny, then drizzle over the top.

10. Leave to set for 10 minutes before slicing into 10 equal slices
and enjoying.

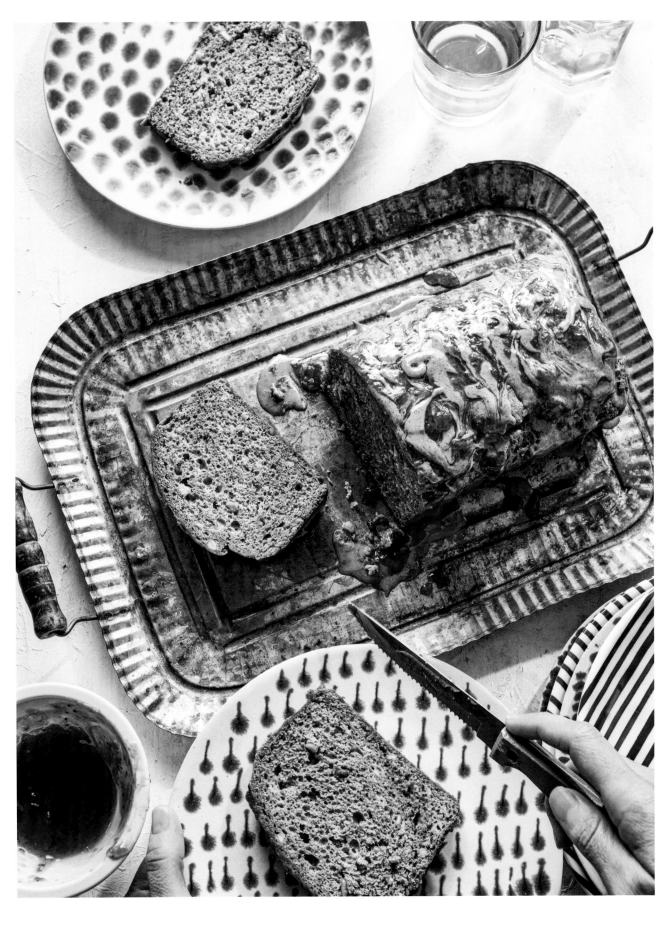

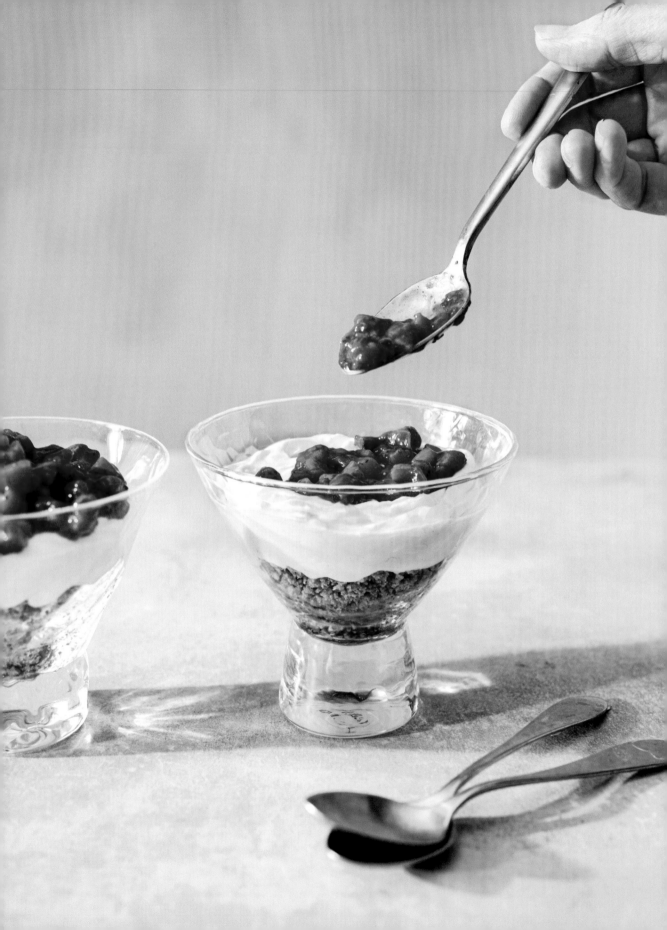

No-bake Strawberry Cheesecakes

MAKES 4 CHEESECAKES

4 reduced-fat digestives, crumbled
¾ tablespoon butter, melted
120g (4oz) light cream cheese
200g (7oz) fat-free Greek yoghurt
3 tablespoons granulated sweetener
1 teaspoon vanilla extract
1 tablespoon lemon juice
a little lemon zest

For the topping:
300g (10oz) frozen strawberries
½ tablespoon granulated sweetener
1½ tablespoons lemon juice
½ tablespoon cornflour (cornstarch)

Variations:
Try different fruit toppings for these, for example banana, kiwi and mandarin oranges (tinned) – you won't need to cook them.

Gluten-free:
Use a gluten-free biscuit of choice.

Swap:
If you prefer you can use maple syrup or honey instead of sweetener, but this will increase the calories.

I have a bit of a weakness for cheesecake – there's just something about that crumbly biscuit base and sweet cream cheese topping. These no-bake strawberry cheesecakes combine cream cheese and Greek yoghurt for a lightened-up version.

1. Crush the digestives and mix with the melted butter.

2. Put into the base of 4 small glasses, pushing down firmly, and refrigerate while you make the topping.

3. Mix the cream cheese until smooth, then add the Greek yoghurt, sweetener, vanilla, lemon juice and zest and mix until combined.

4. Spoon this over the biscuits and put back into the fridge.

5. Put the strawberries, sweetener and lemon juice into a saucepan and heat until the fruit has softened.

6. Mix the cornflour with a little water to make a slurry and add this to the pan, then continue to heat until the mixture is jam-like. Allow to cool, then spoon on top of the cream cheese.

7. Enjoy chilled.

KCALS	**178**
FAT	**5.0g**
SAT FAT	**2.6g**
CARBS	**21.4g**
SUGARS	**12.2g**
FIBRE	**2.0g**
PROTEIN	**10.2g**
SALT	**0.45g**

178 Calories

Chocolate Orange Rice Pudding

SERVES 3

90g (3¼oz) pudding rice,
    rinsed
320ml (11fl oz) water
320ml (11fl oz) 2% milk
    (semi-skimmed)
10g (¼oz) 100% cocoa
    powder
1 vanilla pod, halved (or
    1 teaspoon vanilla extract)
a little orange zest
15g (½oz) milk chocolate
2 tablespoons granulated
    sweetener
1 egg yolk

For the topping:
1 large orange, peeled and
    broken into segments
light aerosol cream (optional)

Dairy-free:
This can be made with
dairy-free milk and
chocolate, but is not quite
as creamy as when you use
regular milk. For the best
result, use cashew milk
if you can get it.

Rice pudding is always a creamy and decadent treat, and this version takes it to a whole other level, perfect for all the chocolate lovers out there. The slight orange flavour in the pudding and the oranges in the topping make it even more decadent.

1. Put the rice into a saucepan with the water, bring to the boil, then cover and simmer until the water has been absorbed. Turn off the heat and leave with the lid on for 10–15 minutes (don't stir). This will continue to cook the rice to perfection.

2. Add the milk, cocoa powder, vanilla, orange zest, milk chocolate and sweetener and stir until creamy, then remove from the heat and quickly stir in the egg yolk.

3. Top with the oranges.

4. Some light aerosol cream is a great addition to the top too, if you like.

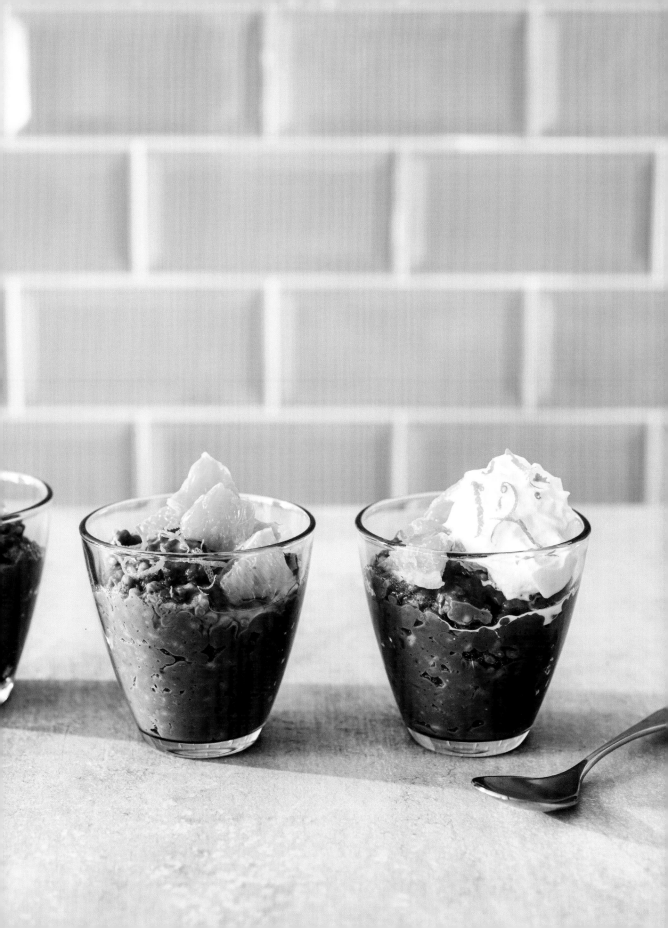

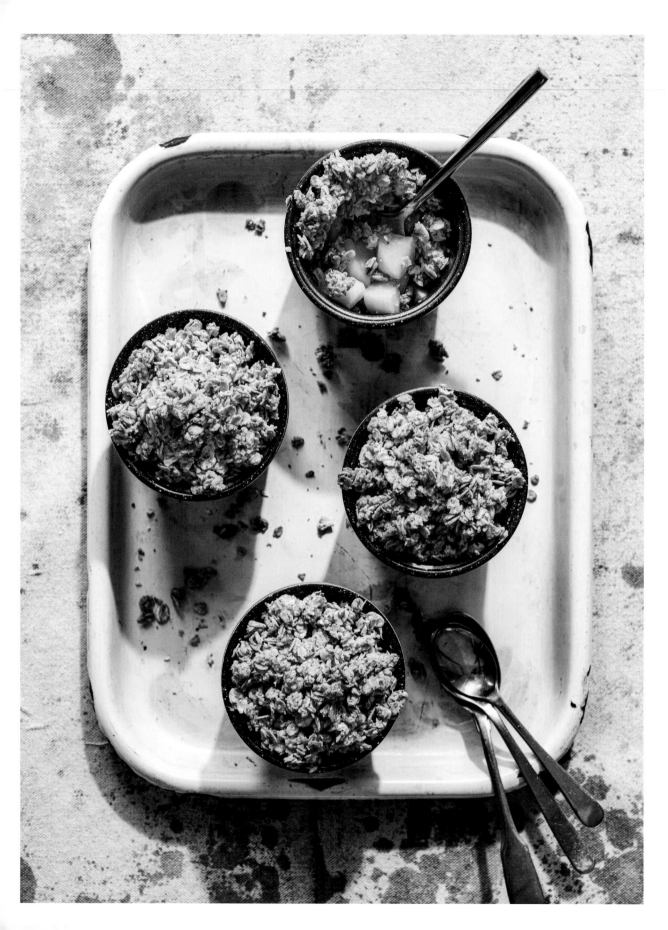

Oaty Apple Crumble

318 Calories

SERVES 4

500g (1lb 2oz) apples, peeled and diced
60ml (2fl oz) apple juice
pinch of ground cinnamon (optional)

For the crumble topping:
160g (6oz) rolled oats
40g (1½oz) Demerara sugar (or brown sugar)
20g (¾oz) butter, softened
1 egg white
cooking oil spray

Dairy-free:
Use dairy-free butter or coconut oil.

Gluten-free:
Use gluten-free oats.

Variation:
Use the oat crumble topping to create different flavours. There are so many options for the fruit – plums, mixed berries, cherries, mango and pineapple, stewed rhubarb, or a combination of any fruits you like.

Lighten the calories:
This recipe makes 4 decent-sized servings. If you want to lower the calories, this can be made in one big dish and will easily serve 6.

Freezing:
Best frozen after step 4. When ready to eat, follow steps 5 and 6, checking the crumbles are hot before serving.

This light apple crumble uses rolled oats for a crunchy golden topping and is a lovely after-dinner treat, served just as it is warm from the oven or with some light cream or custard.

1. Preheat the oven to 190°C/170°C fan/375°F/gas mark 5.

2. Put the apples into a saucepan with the apple juice and cook for a few minutes, until lightly softened. Add a pinch of cinnamon if you like.

3. Divide the apples between 4 round dishes (approx.12cm/5 inches) or one large dish.

4. Put the oats, sugar and softened butter into a bowl and crumble between your fingertips until all combined. Stir in the egg white.

5. Sprinkle over the apples and spray the top with cooking oil.

6. Place in the oven and bake for 30 minutes, until the crumble topping is golden and the apples are really softened.

7. Serve – it's great as it is or with some light aerosol cream or custard.

KCALS	318
FAT	8.2g
SAT FAT	3.3g
CARBS	52.2g
SUGARS	25.3g
FIBRE	4.6g
PROTEIN	6.4g
SALT	0.14g

347
Calories

GF

V

KCALS
347

FAT
11.7g

SAT FAT
1.0g

CARBS
41.7g

SUGARS
39.8g

FIBRE
2.6g

PROTEIN
17.5g

SALT
0.15g

Cinnamon Sugar Pecan-baked Bananas with Greek Yoghurt

SERVES 2

2 ripe bananas (not
  overripe, though)
22 pecan halves, roughly
  chopped
coconut oil spray
2 tablespoons Demerara
  sugar
½ teaspoon ground
  cinnamon
285g (10oz) fat-free
  Greek yoghurt

Dairy-free:
Serve with a dairy-free
yoghurt of your choice.

Variations:
Try different chopped nuts,
or even a crushed biscuit of
your choice, instead of the
pecans.

Sugar swap:
If you prefer to save some
calories you can swap the
Demerara sugar for a brown
granulated sweetener, but
you won't get quite the same
caramelization.

Lighten the calories:
Bananas are quite high
in calories before adding
anything else. If you want
to reduce the calories in
this dessert, enjoy a smaller
serving (½ banana) with
yoghurt.

Buying too many bananas seems to be a weekly occurrence in my household, so when I have some I want to use up, this recipe for baked bananas is a go-to. I love the way the Demerara sugar caramelizes around the pecans to form a yummy topping on the warm baked bananas. Perfect served over Greek yoghurt or with some low-calorie ice cream or frozen yoghurt of your choice.

1. Preheat the oven to 200°C/180°C fan/400°F/gas 6.

2. Peel the bananas and slice them in half lengthways. Place them in an ovenproof baking dish.

3. Put the pecans into a bowl, spray with coconut oil, then add the sugar and cinnamon and toss until the pecans are all coated.

4. Sprinkle the nuts over the top of the bananas and spray the top with coconut oil.

5. Bake for 15–20 minutes, until golden and caramelized.

6. Serve with the Greek yoghurt.

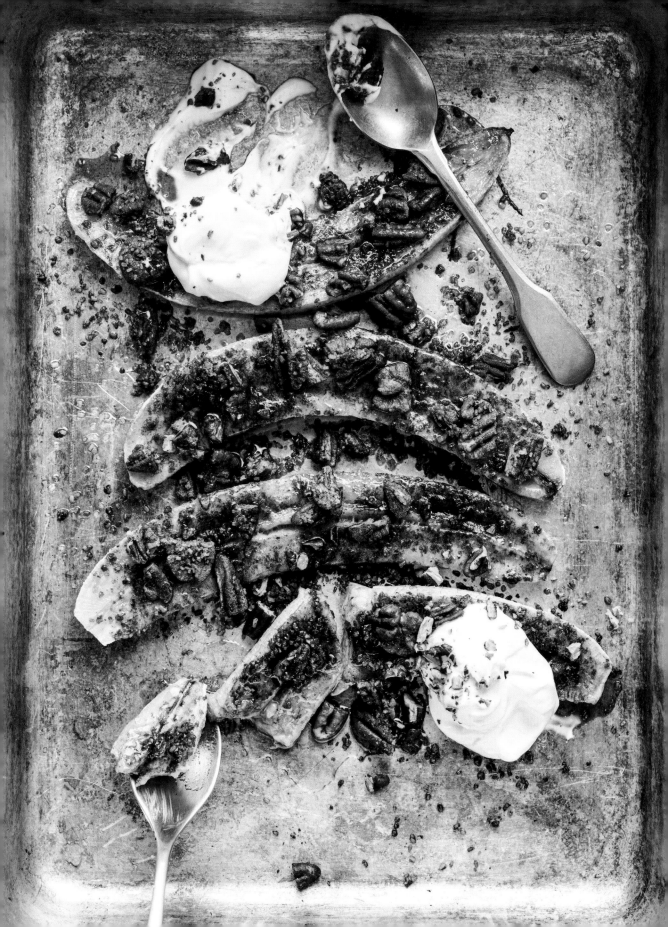

Index

Acknowledgements

I never imagined I would be writing an acknowledgements page! It seems crazy and surreal to me that you love my recipes so much that you would want to buy my book.

I have been asked several times to write a book, but resisted for various reasons. 2020, however, was incredibly hard in many ways and I realized that life is too short to miss out – so now feels like the right time. A massive thanks to Hodder & Stoughton, Yellow Kite Books and Mobius, without whom this book would never have been possible. And a very special thank you to Lauren Whelan, who regularly checked in on me to see if I would change my mind until one day I did.

When it came to writing the book, I was anxious about how I would manage with deadlines and throwing myself into 100 brand new recipes, especially in the middle of a strict Covid lockdown. But my husband Gavin and my children Isaac and Felicity were supportive and encouraging from the start. The kids played a huge part in deciding which recipes made it into the book. My husband took over the website and was on the receiving end of all my stress, while I threw myself into cooking, testing and retesting sometimes 6+ recipes a day. I could never have done it without the support of the three of them.

Once the recipes were done came the excitement of seeing everything come together. The photoshoot was done in London by the amazing and talented photographers Liz and Max Haarala Hamilton, the beautiful props and styling by the lovely Jen Kay, and the cooking and styling of the recipes by Rosie Reynolds and Aya Nishimura, brilliantly assisted by Hanna Miller and Troy Willis. Unfortunately I couldn't be with them in person because of travel restrictions, but it was fun joining in over Zoom most days to see my recipes cooked, styled, photographed and coming to life on my computer screen.

Thanks also to Nathan Burton for revamping the Slimming Eats logo, and for the amazing design and layouts.

A special thank you to Kerry Torrens, who made sure every single recipe has accurate nutritional info so that the recipes are suitable for whatever healthy eating plan you are following. And to copy-editor Annie Lee, for ensuring my garbled instructions are readable and coherent.

I know I mentioned her before, but really I can't thank Lauren Whelan (associate publisher at Yellow Kite) enough. When she first contacted me about doing a book, it was a definite no from me, but she never gave up. Persistent but never pushy, she made me believe in myself and the little website I had created. So thank you, Lauren.

I also have to thank the lovely Isabel Gonzalez-Prendergast (project editor) for always being so patient with my constant string of emails and queries. I am quite a worrier and really like everything to be perfect, and she was the one who answered my concerns and queries, always reassuring me (I did warn you in advance what I am like).

To Giuliana Caranante at Mobius for handling the North American market and making it possible to see my book on the shelves here in Canada. To Sahini Bibi for marketing and for all the stuff behind the scenes in getting my book out there, and to Jenny Platt for the publicity.

A special thank you to my friends Clare and Kerry, for being there for me day and night and for providing emotional support and encouragement when needed. Also to my lifelong friends Nicky, Nicola and Kate for their continued friendship and support.

To my lovely neighbour and good friend Kathy, for dragging me out for coffee as an escape when necessary. We definitely need one of our shopping trips as soon as we can, or maybe one of our nights in the garden doing cartwheels.

A massive thank you to Moira, Claire, Steph and Andra, for always being around as extra eyes on my Facebook group and for giving huge support and help to my readers.

Thanks to my dad, Peter (hope the £25k was worth it!), for introducing me to so many different cuisines from a young age, which definitely influenced my love of food.

Thanks to my mum, Frances, who sadly passed away in 2018. I know she would be incredibly proud of what I have achieved and would be shouting out to anyone and everyone in her little home town in Ireland that her daughter has a book out.

To my father-in-law, Colin, and late mother-in-law, Dot, for all their love and their support for Slimming Eats over the years.

And thanks to all my friends and family who have given their support – I am so happy to be able to share this special moment with you all.

Lastly and most importantly, to my readers – those who have supported me from the start and those who have discovered me along the way. Thank you for buying this book. It is your encouragement and support over the years that has kept me doing what I do. There is nothing more rewarding for me than seeing you enjoying my creations and sharing your kind words about how my recipes help you on your healthy eating journey, whether it's through a comment on my website, on social media or through an email. I will continue creating recipes for however long you want to keep cooking them. None of this would be possible without you. I hope you enjoy this cookbook. I've tried my best to ensure it has something for everyone.

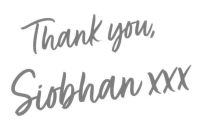

Thank you,
Siobhan xxx

First published in Great Britain in 2021 by Yellow Kite
An imprint of Hodder & Stoughton
An Hachette UK company

1

A CIP catalogue record for this title is available from the British Library

Hardback ISBN 978 1 529 377415
eBook ISBN 978 1 529 377422

Associate Publisher: Lauren Whelan
Project Editor: Isabel Gonzalez-Prendergast
Designer: Nathan Burton
Photography: Liz & Max Haarala Hamilton
Food Stylists: Rosie Reynolds & Aya Nishimura
Props Stylist: Jen Kay
Senior Production Controller: Diana Talyanina

Colour origination by Alta Image London
Printed and bound in Canada by Friesens

Hodder & Stoughton policy is to use papers that are natural, renewable and recyclable products
and made from wood grown in sustainable forests. The logging and manufacturing processes
are expected to conform to the environmental regulations of the country of origin.

Yellow Kite
Hodder & Stoughton Ltd
Carmelite House
50 Victoria Embankment
London
EC4Y 0DZ

www.yellowkitebooks.co.uk
www.hodder.co.uk

Notes
The information and references contained herein are for informational purposes only. They are designed
to support, not replace, any ongoing medical advice given by a healthcare professional and should not be construed as
the giving of medical advice nor relied upon as a basis for any decision or action. Readers should consult their doctor
before altering their diet, particularly if they are on a set diet prescribed by their doctor or dietician.

The calorie count for each recipe is an estimate only and may vary depending on the brand of ingredients used, and due to the
natural biological variations in the composition of foods such as meat, fish, fruit and vegetables. It does not include the nutritional
content of garnishes or any optional accompaniments recommended for taste/serving in the ingredients list